MW00803097

AUTOBIOLOGY OF A VET

John Sauvage

First published 2021
Published by GB Publishing Org
Copyright © John Phillip Sauvage, BVetMed, BA, CertSAC, MRCVS
All rights reserved

ISBNs:
978-1-912576-28-9 (hardback)
978-1-912576-29-6 (paperback)
978-1-912576-30-2 (eBook)
978-1-912576-31-9 (Kindle)

Cover Design © 2021 Mary Pargeter Design

For more photographs and information relevant to this book, please go to
www.johnsauvageautobiology.com

A catalogue record of the printed book is available from
the British Library

GB Publishing Org
www.gbpublishing.co.uk

*Dedicated to my wife Sandra
and all the family*

*With thanks and apologies to all the characters
and animals, none of whom is a figment of my imagination;
all are truly represented to the best of my recollection*

*Thanks to David Ritchie for his help
with editing and getting the book to this stage*

We all know what an "autobiography" is but what is
an "autobiology"? It seemed a great title for a vet's life story.
Biology is the study of life, so John made this word up since animals
and plants are so intricately tied up with his life both studying and as
a veterinary surgeon, as well as his hobbies of gardening
and playing lawn tennis.

CONTENTS

INTRODUCTION

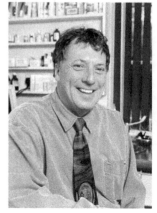

"How did I get here?" to paraphrase David Byrne, is a long story but one worth recording (I hope) before it is too late.

Nobody knows how much time they have and perhaps I have already had more than my share. As Mr Byrne and his *Talking Heads* band says, it is by watching the days go by and for me it is time to record how I ended up in a beautiful house with a beautiful wife.

There I was in the great hall at the Royal Veterinary College (RVC) in Camden Town. The giant gilded portrait of George III whose reign the college was founded in was looking down on me and, more relevant, so was the President of the Royal College of Veterinary Surgeons (RCVS). It was April 1973 and, in the hall, seated alongside me were the rest of my final year, apart from the unlucky few who had failed their final exams.

I clearly remember what Mr Alasdair Steele-Bodger (the RCVS President) said to us before we were officially allowed to practise the art and science of veterinary surgery. I was the exception in the group in that I had special permission from the college and had been allowed to start practice work on April the first.

He told us about what would now be recognised as the triage system. He said there were three types of sick animals. The first group, he continued, would luckily get better whatever and almost despite what we did. The third group would sadly die whatever we did, and it was our duty to make that death as humane as possible. In the middle, he said, there is a small group who with all the expertise we had gleaned would live, but without it would die.

He went on to discuss acute and chronic disease saying that chronic disease was long term and required on-going assistance and probably on-going therapy, but acute disease if treated promptly could end up with a complete cure. He also warned about the most severe form of acute disease, so called per-acute disease. This would require the utmost aggressive therapy if it were not to end in death.

So, the take-home message, or rather the take-back-to-our-practices message, was to do what we could for the small group that without our help would go on to chronic disease and suffering or death.

Little did I realise that the improvements in veterinary medicine and surgery over the next fifty years would increase substantially that small middle group.

This is my story and to some little extent my walk-on part in that bigger picture.

1

BATTLE OF BRITAIN DAY

So how did I get here? I was born on 15th September, 1949, the ninth anniversary of the Battle of Britain and my battle with life was just beginning. It was a dark rainy night in Streatham, south-west London, and my mother always said I was in a hurry and her original and main reason for this was my speedy unannounced arrival.

Suddenly I started to arrive, and my mother yelled to my gran – my father always worked nights – to quickly get a midwife. As the nearest telephone box was about three hundred yards up the road my gran grabbed her hat and coat and fumbled in her purse for four pennies to put in the box and press button A if connected, B if not to get your 4d back. My mother screamed at her with broken waters and my big head already emerging that this was an emergency and she should dial 999.

My gran nodded and ran out of our two-bedroomed downstairs flat, returning a few minutes later with a "midwife". Only it was not a midwife, it was the local police constable (PC) on his beat who had seen my gran rushing up the street. I do not know if PCs were any older then than now or even look any older, but I suspect he was as shocked as everyone else to see me greeting the world.

Anyway, he did a great job and I arrived. Several years later the PC came round for tea; he was pleased to have been promoted to sergeant and was still proud of his midwifery experience. I must have been about four because I remember he showed me his dark wooden heavy truncheon and whistle and obviously enjoyed chatting to my mother. The police visit was not my earliest childhood recollection and in case you are asking I have no idea if my dad knew about the policeman's

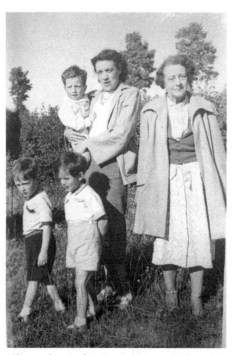

The author in his mother's arms, alongside his English grandmother, elder brother Tony (in front of mother) with cousin Rod next to him

visit or visits, but I am sure they were innocent as it was after all the 1950s.

My earliest childhood memory was being in a great big chariot of a pram. It was the same perambulator my elder brother and cousin had shared and the same one used by me, then my younger cousin and younger brother. Before you say impossible to remember being in a pram, I suspect they were used on kids for a lot longer and older then.

I also think I remember falling out of it and dangling by one strap over the side, then pulling the pram on top of me. My Aunt Joan later told the story in full. Apparently, she took me to the local park and only fixed the harness on one side; I fell over the edge dangling by the one strap and then the pram gently tipped over onto me. I am not sure if that is a first-hand memory or my aunt's tale recycled but I do remember being in that pram.

I also clearly remember my father taking us to The Mall to see the newly-crowned Queen go by in a carriage so that would have been 2nd June 1953 and I would have been heading for my fourth birthday the following September.

My mother and Aunt Joan had always been involved with dogs. My maternal grandfather had been the kennel man for the Maharajah of Jind in India after the first war and in about 1952 they started getting involved with miniature dachshunds. It was this interest in dachshund showing that led them and me to Crufts in that same year, 1953, and I made the national papers standing with my miniature dachshund in the kids' class next to a St Bernard and the headline "A dog and a dog's dinner". I even have a press cutting in French. Perhaps this was my destiny to grow up with dogs and make my living from them like my mother, aunt and grandfather.

2

PRIMARY SCHOOL

I was playing in the front garden defeating an invisible enemy with a wooden sword when my mother told me the next day would be my first day of school.

After walking to Hitherfield Primary with my mother the following day, there are only two distant memories of my whole time in the infant department. The first was learning to read. I was certainly slow at both reading and writing and struggled to keep up. This was made worse by poor attendance exacerbated by poor health. I was quite asthmatic with wheezing in the summer due to pollen allergies and coughing in the winter due to secondary bronchitis.

The asthma was controlled using a delicate glass inhaler with a pump bottom that would deliver an inhaled dose of what I think was a salbutamol or other bronchodilator liquid turned into a spray. It was certainly delicate, and I broke it at least twice a year, having to spend several wheezy hunched-up days and nights waiting for a replacement. In hindsight I suspect the dog dander and smoke from my mother's cigarettes as well as fumes from paraffin heaters did not help.

I never took a moment to consider car exhausts because we did not have a car and neither did anyone else in the street but the coalman certainly delivered to most houses nearby. For the last twenty years I have been having annual flu vaccination and that has certainly controlled the annual bronchitis attacks and brings me to my other infant school memory, that of polio vaccination.

I had seen kids in leg irons and remember my mother telling me some children even needed iron lungs, whatever they were, after catching polio. So, I was happy to go along with my mother's rule of not taking my brother or me to public swimming pools for fear of catching the 'virus'. At this time, my mother regularly had her dogs vaccinated with "Epivax", the first dog distemper vaccine, so when she said there was a polio vaccine clinic at the school and that she had signed me up for it, I was to say the least worried as I had seen the dogs inoculated with a big silver syringe and an exceptionally large, even for little puppies, silver needle.

I remember joining the queue and waiting in line in the playground with knees knocking just below my little shorts. After the children entered the building none came out and my fear grew.

Imagine my relief when it was my turn to just be given a sugar lump to eat. This vaccine business was a "piece of cake" or better still a sugar lump. No wonder I remembered.

My promotion to the Junior School happened in 1957 and my memories are how kind the headmaster Mr Henley-Jones was, how nice all the lady teachers were, especially Miss Disney who had apparently spent a lot of time in the Sudan, but everyone's favourite was Mr Veal, a charming man with a love of sport and an infectious enthusiasm for life. Probably a good teacher but such a sadistic disciplinarian was Slipper Scott: he took great pride and enjoyment in beating boys.

There was a school code of personal credits and debits, both of which involved announcements in front of the whole school in assembly. If Scott heard that a pupil in his class got a personal debit, he would slipper them for good measure that same morning as if public humiliation were not enough.

I managed one personal credit for learning and reciting the 23rd Psalm in the headmaster's study, but my backside became a target for Scott's slipper only once and the injustice hurt more than the smack on my backside. It was not for earning a personal debit but for breaking a classroom rule.

The rule was that nobody could go out of the prefab classroom window on to the grassland behind. I clearly remember several of the girls in the class distressed when I walked in because of an injured blackbird outside the window so I simply climbed out the window and passed it to them, then climbed back in. Mr Scott walked in and immediately spotted small muddy footprints from the window across the room. When he asked who had been out of the window, I immediately owned up, telling him exactly what had happened. He slippered me before dealing with the bird as the "rules are the rules". My first real animal rescue had not gone too well.

More later in my story on my views on corporal punishment in schools but I think the education system is better without it and the personal debit and personal credit system did not need amplifying with physical abuse.

Two of my closest friends there, Colin and Martin, are now back in touch thanks to the Internet. Colin had the same birthday as me and I was disappointed at the time to find out he was older than me – born in the morning. Now I am pleased to say I am the youngest of the three of us.

The greatest highlight of my time at Hitherfield was the school journey to Hopton-on-Sea in Norfolk, in which most of the school spent a week away taking over a holiday camp. What a fun-packed week it was. I remember a boat trip to the Norfolk Broads when I saw my first heron. A magnificent bird that never fails to impress me even when they are still after the fish in my ponds.

We had a trip to Norwich Castle, Colman's Mustard Factory, a trip to Lowestoft watching kippers smoked, and Norwich Cathedral. The grave of Nurse Edith Cavell, shot by the Germans in 1915 for helping allied prisoners to escape, was vivid as I had seen the film about her. She has a statue just off Trafalgar Square opposite the National Portrait Gallery. The biggest let-down of the week was the cancellation of the trip to Smith's Crisps factory.

Two memorable events on the trip were a game of proper hard ball cricket umpired by Mr Veal. I am told this was a trial for the school team but as usual I did not make the team. I have recently been given a photo of the school football team at the time and I am certainly not in it.

The other highlight was an evening after the return from a trip when I was called by a group of excited kids to see an amazing site.

Behind the chalets was what looked like a giant dead rat, but I was told it was a coypu. A burial party was soon organised, and he was named Roland Rat. I had nothing to do with the burial and would now warn the children that did deal with him that rats and coypu's carry leptospirosis, a bacterium that causes Weil's Disease in humans and is an essential component in modern dog vaccines. These days there would be an uproar if 11-year-old kids on a school trip were unsupervised and allowed to expose themselves to such a nasty disease.

During my last year at Hitherfield I was in Mr Veal's class and he put newspaper cuttings on the class noticeboard. One I remember was a headline about the Duke of Edinburgh on a tiger shoot in January 1961: there were several pictures of him riding an elephant with the Queen and posing with the body of a tiger he had personally shot. British and Indian politicians were outraged and so was my primary school class. Ironically, I have since found out that he became the President of the British branch of the World Wildlife Fund in the same year.

3

COMPREHENSIVE SCHOOL

I failed the eleven plus exams, though not by much, the primary school headmaster told my parents. I can even remember one of the questions was, "Which of these English cities has a port?" London was on the list and as it was inland, I stupidly assumed it could not have a port. Thousands of dockers would have laughed at my ignorance. My mates in the playground afterwards certainly did when I told them I had not included my hometown of London in the list.

So, it was Tulse Hill Comprehensive for me: a giant seven-storey new-build trying to educate more than two thousand boys all at the same time.

It had only opened about four years before and my elder brother Tony was already there. He was a couple of years behind the most famous old boy of the school, Ken Livingstone.

I was saddened that most of my friends went on to local posh grammar schools such as Alleyn's and even Dulwich College and other local private schools.

I was twelve or thirteen when I decided I wanted to be a vet. My mother bred several litters a year and there were always little dachshunds running about. The breed is not particularly good at whelping, especially the miniature variety which must be under 11 pounds (5kg) when adult. One night I stayed up all night doing a shift of overseeing labour and nest building; then, when proper straining occurred and a water bag appeared, calling my mother who had caught up on some much-needed sleep. Within twenty minutes of her joining me the first puppy was born. It was wrapped in a membrane of fluid and looked like a 'bubble-gum bubble' before the membrane burst and a little puppy was quickly forced out without needing any help. Half an hour later a second puppy was born; unlike the first one which was head first, this came bottom first but no problems as dachshunds have such little legs. The last puppy was born head first within the hour. Then the dam cleaned up the afterbirths and all the puppies were quickly suckling a very contented and proud mum.

I then went to bed, but I remember the vet coming the next morning. A lovely man called Frank Beattie; he was a very skilled practitioner whose family still runs a travel grant in his memory through the British Small Animal Veterinary Association. He came to check the litter when it arrived, and I remember even did a caesarean on several of my mother's dogs with fantastic results. Just a few of these home calls and I decided on my future career. Just the minor issue of getting to veterinary college.

I was in the fourth academic stream which meant I had to do metalwork, woodwork, bricklaying, plumbing and plastering as well as academic subjects including Latin. I absolutely hated the practical parts gearing me towards an apprenticeship in the trades and when after two years only the top three classes kept on with Latin my parents and I argued with the school to spare me the trade work but I had to give up Latin. Luckily, the school agreed, and my curriculum focused on the sciences but sadly now I wish I had also paid a little more attention in those classes as I lack many of the basic DIY skills everyone needs.

All fifteen-year-olds in the school were tested for TB using a Tuberculin skin test and those like me with a negative were then given the BCG vaccine – this was also a painless skin injection. The level of TB in both people and cattle was going down in the country at the time thanks to the human testing and vaccination programme and the cattle testing and slaughter policy of any infected herds.

As I say, I focused on the sciences for my O levels studying physics and chemistry but instead of standard biology I did a specialist nursing O level course on Human Anatomy, Physiology and Hygiene, known as Human AP&H. I found this extremely interesting and so helpful with my first two years at veterinary college which involved in-depth anatomy, which is the study of the structure of animals, and physiology, the study of how they function. I also had to cover one arts subject and chose economic history as well as English and maths and compulsory religious knowledge. As I keep saying, for various reasons I was always slow at learning but once the principle was grasped, I really understood complicated concepts. As a dog trainer once said to me, Labradors are quick to learn and quick to forget but Golden Retrievers are slow to learn but never forget. I sometimes wonder if I am the unlucky cross of the two: slow to learn and quick to forget!

I was always a bit of a joker in class and my art teacher the year before I gave up the subject said in my school report, "A bit silly." My sense of humour finally got me into trouble with my physics teacher. He was leaning over an electric heater circuit demonstrating how a wire turns red hot when a current is passed through it and I said, much to the amusement of the class, "Your beard is alight, Sir." He jumped up and was not amused to find I was joking and I was sent to the Head of Science. Both he and I thought I would just get a reprimand as I was certainly working hard at the time. To my surprise, the head of department wanted to cane me, and I did what very few did in this time of corporal punishment: I refused to bend over. Was its fear of the physical punishment or the burning sense of injustice from the blackbird incident? I was certainly more scared of the consequences of my refusal than the potential pain, but stubbornly stuck to my refusal. As a result, I was excluded from the physics class for the rest of the term and had to work under the direct supervision of the Head of Science who was also a physics teacher. So refusing the cane was a strange but effective way to get one-on-one tuition from one of the best teachers in the school.

Anyway, at some time after this sad incident and because of my exclusion from the class, somewhere around fourteen years of age I got a hunger to learn. I clearly remember a rainy dark winter night when there was nothing to do but my physics homework and once that was done I read a bit of the textbook and ended up reading the whole book. It was the same with the other science subjects and social and economic history seemed just as logical.

I was not the only lad in the O level science classes who wanted to be a vet. My best friend at the time was a lad called Mike. He was brighter than I was but was told to leave school by his father and get a real job. In no time he was working in a baker's and we sadly lost touch until recently when again, thanks to the Internet, he contacted me.

When it came to the exams (no continual assessment in those days) I did not do very well in my mocks so started waking up in the middle of the night when the house was perfectly quiet and studying. I made the logical conclusion to give up on French after a shocking French mock failure, or more likely the school decided to save the entrance fee and not enter me. The focus worked and I passed O levels well enough to do the three sciences of physics, chemistry and zoology at A level. The zoology allowed me to again miss out on botany, the study of plants and the other half of life.

By this time, I had decided I wanted to be a vet but my career adviser at school had other ideas saying that I would be lucky to get into university let alone vet school and would be far better off doing a teaching degree or at best studying for a degree in physics. He did, however, reassure me that it did not matter that I had given up Latin but to get to a vet school I would need an O level language such as French and many would not accept Human AP&H and would require O level biology. So, I ignored his guidance and applied to the six veterinary colleges in the UK at the time: London, Glasgow, Cambridge, Bristol, Liverpool, Edinburgh. There was also Dublin in the Republic of Ireland but I was only allowed to apply to six.

I also revisited French but again soon gave up before the exam, but was more successful getting O level biology during the first year of my A level studies, mainly by swatting up on the life-cycle of the cabbage white butterfly outside the exam room five minutes before the exam. How lucky was that. I did do a little botanical study as well for that examination, but the majority of my plant knowledge is from learning about poisonous plants and arable crops at college or from my much later interest in gardening. I promptly got three rejections from Glasgow, Edinburgh and Bristol, an interview from Cambridge (which if successful meant an entry exam) and two so-called 'waiting lists' from London and Liverpool. Waiting list meant the university might make an offer depending on exam results. It was now too late to apply to Dublin.

Enough of my academic career at Tulse Hill, what about my life there?

It was such a massive school and I was there for seven years, starting as a raw first year wandering around what appeared to me at the time to be a glass skyscraper, trying to find the correct classroom out of seven floors with over thirty rooms on each corridor. The glass staircases looking out over the playground probably gave me my fear of heights. I still have nightmares of being on the school roof, looking over the edge and toppling to the hard concrete seven floors down. Not that I ever went on the roof! The art, science and workshop facilities were second to none and we were transported out to Epping Playing Fields every Wednesday for sport, but again I did not make it into any teams, although I did participate in football in the winter, athletics in the summer and even tried my hand at squash. I started playing tennis towards the end of my time at the school but only on local park courts and not through the school and was never coached until later life and still love to play.

There was also an active Army Cadet Force and Air Training Corps, the ACF and the ATC. I followed my brother into the ATC and spent time on the rifle ranges of Bisley and Pirbright and summer camps at various RAF bases such as RAF Ternhill near Market Drayton between the ages of eleven and fifteen. I was certainly given good weapons training which came in handy when having to handle guns for humane killing in my chosen career. I also went for an acrobatic flight in a trainer de Havilland Chipmunk. I had no fear if during a loop I could look at the floor of the aircraft and that was down for me. My fear of flying came later.

I will always remember the adage that the gun is always loaded and the safety catch off, whatever anyone tells you. The highlight of my time in the ATC was the Ten Tors. This involved trekking over Dartmoor for 48 hours in groups of six. If all six in the party completed the exercise, an individual medal and certificate was awarded; if one or more dropped out, a certificate only was awarded. Our team leader Pat was a brilliant navigator and led from the front. He was a corporal, we were just cadets.

Most of us had been on many practice treks out into the Kent countryside at weekends, both officially with the cadets and organised by our leader. We were the under sixteen years-old team and we were officially meant to be over fifteen to enter. I certainly was underage, but nobody checked. I say most of us did all the training but there was one big, tall member of the team, Len, who did not make it to many of the training days. The Dartmoor weekend finally arrived, and we were at the start of day one. My elder brother had done the exercise the previous year but not all his team completed, and he was doing it again but the over 16 course this time. Unlike us, his team decided to carry tents, but we decided to travel light with just cold food and ground sheets which meant a bit of a gamble with the unpredictable Dartmoor weather. The course was meant to be just under 40 miles, meaning we should cover half of that a day. Because it was called Ten Tors and by mid-morning we had been to five checkpoints and up and down at least five Tors, I was bubbly and optimistic that we had cracked the exercise. I was most disappointed to find out there were many more than ten checkpoints and we certainly went up and down more than ten of the famous hills.

It did not take long before the real lack of fitness, both mental and physical, of my tall friend began to show. He was lagging and complaining his feet hurt. As the afternoon wore on it seemed we had walked miles without a checkpoint, and we were off the moor having crossed a cattle bridge and the "You Are Now leaving Dartmoor" sign was far behind us. This did not bother us because the route often weaved in and out of the National Park boundary. It was only then that the team leader and his assistant navigator Colin told us we were lost. We walked on and found a village marked on the map and discovered we were at least three miles off course. I was good at map reading but was a bit baffled by bearings and spent most of my time chatting to our lanky "Tail End Charlie" Len to keep his spirits up and ensure we all finished with medals.

We headed back to the moor and finally got to the next checkpoint at the top of a Tor, the tallest and most exhausting climb of the day I remember. The squaddies at the checkpoint suggested we quit as it would be dark soon and we would have too much to do the next day. All of us, including my very tired friend Len, were determined to carry on as if there were no more navigational errors we could make up the lost time. We managed another level checkpoint, had some hot tea there and were on our way to the next one when we decided to stop for the night. We did not light a fire, had our cold bully rations and looked at our ground sheets and wondered what we should do.

It was logical that we paired up with one fellow's groundsheet on the ground and the others on top of the pair of us. I partnered up with Colin; we had taken off our boots and it seemed heavenly and warm with an extra pair of socks on, but the temperature quickly dropped and the air was damp. I have never been so cold as I was that night or cuddled a man so closely just to share warmth with the groundsheet over our heads and a woolly hat pulled over my face. Apart from the woolly hats we were cheek to cheek with legs and arms wrapped around each other We did not sleep but shivered the night away with chattering teeth. In the early hours of the morning, we packed away our groundsheet into our rucksacks, put our boots on by torchlight and were ready to go at the first crack of dawn – still shivering.

The day was the longest I have ever known, and I was getting further and further behind with Len and, the truth be told, I was exhausted. At the next checkpoint we were told how far behind the other teams we were, and the retirement option was given again. Trying to keep up with the others I suggested we sing like we did on some of our marches through Kent in training and we burst into "It's a long way to Tipperary" and every other army, pop or rugby song we knew the words of, or thought we did and the group's morale lifted.

It did not take long before the sight of a few more hills dampened us. Then I looked behind and saw Len sitting on a rock. I went back to him and he said he'd had enough and wanted to quit. The others were by now 300 yards ahead. I waved to them to stop and they waited but did not come back. The thought of an extra 600 yards was too much for even them as well. I did not sit down on the rock next to him but leant over him. I knew if I sat down, I too would quit. I gently reminded him of the medal, and he said he did not care. Then I shouted at him and he started to cry. I pulled his arm with tears running down my cheeks. Was I crying too or was it windy? I screamed at him, "We have all got to do this or we won't get a medal." I grabbed his arm and pulled, and he reluctantly stood up. "You won't tell the others I cried, will you?" he asked. "Not if you complete the Ten Tors," I replied. We slowly caught the others up and trekked on, sometimes singing but usually lost in our own thoughts.

I asked how many checkpoints left and was disheartened by the reply. Then about three in the afternoon Len looked at me and said he wanted to quit again but as he did not sit down I just chatted to him, but a half hour later, with the others well ahead of us, he was starting to take off his rucksack and beginning to sit down. I rushed behind him and firmly kicked his squatting backside. "Don't you dare sit down!" I hollered and to my surprise he trudged on and I kept chatting to him. We remained a good 100 yards behind the others and finally got to the finish. We climbed into a single decker bus to get us back to the campsite, but I was asleep before the driver started the engine.

At the campsite I was reunited with my brother whose team had dropped out early in the second day. "Our course is much longer," he said, and "we were carrying tents", not knowing how many extra miles we had done. The presentations were made, and I put my medal and certificate in my tent and we all went for a meal and a drink. Len was grinning from ear to ear and was so proud of himself and his big

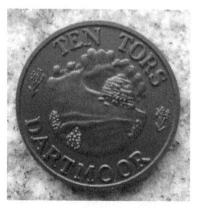

The Dartmoor Ten Tors medal

blisters. His blisters were bigger than mine but so were his feet.

Then disaster struck. I got back to my tent and found it had been raided and my medal stolen. Obviously, somebody who had completed the course but without a full team had taken my medal and all I had to show for completing the Ten Tors was a certificate and my blisters.

This story eventually has a happy ending as just last year my wife and daughter found a Ten Tors Medal on eBay and bought it for me, so I have the medal at home at last.

I was active in the year drama competition in 1964 and got a part in the house play. It was an improvisation, and we did not win the competition but ours was filmed by the BBC during rehearsals and televised, meaning my parents got a cheque for three guineas (£3.3s), so perhaps rather than my later script writing exploits in which I got a better fee but no credit in the titles, this was my 15 minutes of fame. Perhaps somewhere in the BBC archives is the recorded film sequence, "The Sound of Voices:5124/2389 Working Title-The Long Weekend". I doubt it but I still have the letter from them.

I also did several jobs, starting with a paper round which I was doing in 1963. I not only remember exactly what I was doing the night the world heard of the assassination of President Kennedy, I read every newspaper's version of what happened the next morning as I delivered the sad, bad news through the letterboxes. Kennedy was a hero of mine as I remember being in the playground at school the year before when we were looking at the sky expecting Russian Missiles over London any minute and he had stopped that happening with his handling of the Cuban Missile crisis.

Another holiday job I had was at the Whiteley's store in Bayswater.

I spent several school holidays there and one of the part-time workers was a second-year student at the Royal Veterinary College, so I had lots of questions for him. One I particularly remember was, "Why do dogs bleed at the point of mating and ovulation whereas women bleed at the opposite point in the cycle furthest from ovulation?" He explained that a woman's uterus was shedding its wall that had been ready for foetal implantation, but the bitch was simply undergoing vaginal changes, first bleeding and then producing a thicker membrane layer to accommodate mating. This completely cleared up a major biological question my Human AP&H O level syllabus had not clarified for me.

The other memorable event that happened involved a human skin specialist. I mentioned my health had not been good as a little kid and before my asthma I suffered with eczema where my skin got sore and itchy. It was so bad at one stage that I was hospitalised pre-school, so must have been around four years old. In hospital I was put in a cot and covered in a blanket that made me even more irritated, so I came out worse than I went in. My father heard that one of the diners in the nightclub where he was a waiter at the time (I think the Café de Paris?), was a dermatologist, so asked for his help. As a result I was recruited on a trial at no cost to my father and visited Harley Street weekly to see this dermatologist and take part in a special light ray trial.

Anyway, to bring the story up to speed, I was working in the shoe department at Whiteley's when an incredibly old man limped in and sat down. He wanted a pair of brown brogue shoes and I served him. He paid by American Express credit card – almost unheard of at the time as everybody paid by cash or occasionally a cheque. But how lucky was this, I saw his name on the card and knew I recognised him but now I knew where and how. He was the Harley Street dermatologist, Dr Hassen. I told him my name and he immediately remembered how my father had insisted on talking to him. I thanked him for curing me and for all his help *pro bono*. He said, "My dear boy, I was so pleased I could help. The ultraviolet light ray was rubbish but didn't the cortisone cream do the trick – I never thought that would work."

He asked what I was doing and told him I wanted to be a vet and we chatted about his work and he told me he was long retired and limped off giving the distinct impression he was either incredibly pleased with his new shoes or proud to have encountered one of his successful cases many years after retirement, proving the benefits of corticosteroid cream, a product he had pioneered in the fifties.

4

HOW DID I GET HERE?

So here I was at Tulse Hill in my final year of A Levels. I had become a school prefect and then Head of House which meant I not only had access to the sixth form common room but also a room for just the six heads of house and the head boy. There was a chess set in the room and that is where it all nearly went wrong. I spent more and more time playing chess and less studying. One day I was in the middle of a game when a friend came in and told me I had better get to my zoology class or else. I rushed up the five flights of stairs ten minutes late for the lesson after which the Master who became a good friend warned me to either give up chess or give up my ambition to be a vet.

I took his advice and have hardly played since. A similar Bridge school at the vet college led to a friend failing first year exams and having to leave.

It was probably this one-track attitude that made me fail my Cambridge vet school interview. The interview did not go well. I did not realise that it was the individual colleges that do the interview, not the vet school, and when the panel were asking questions, none about veterinary matters to probe how rounded I was, I kept bringing the topic back to how hard I was studying. A memorable line from obviously an angler on the panel was, "So I see you like fishing?"

"When did you last fish?" My answer of not for two years went down badly. "Not a very keen angler," was his riposte. "You like tennis, do you play for a club?" "No, I just play in the park courts," was not a winning reply.

"I see you play chess." "Yes, but I've given it up so I can study for my A levels," was another place-losing response.

So that just left me with no conditional offers and just Liverpool or London who would not offer me a place until after my exam results were out.

The exams went well. I was so lucky because the Science A level sixth form classes were so small with five or six in each class and the teachers were of such high calibre because the Comprehensive system was in its infancy and they were educational idealists. My physics master even had a PhD. I was in the right place at the correct time. I had better one-on-one tuition than any private or other school in the land, including Dulwich College or Alleyne's.

I was so pleased to receive my grades: B in physics, B in zoology and C in chemistry. These days would need straight A+ grades but August 1968 was a long time ago and I would like to think A levels were much harder then. A few nail-biting days later I got a letter from the Royal Veterinary College in London offering me a place.

So, that is how I got to vet college, but how did I get here in the broader sense? How did my Belgian father meet my English mother and how did they get to Streatham in the suburbs of London? I do not know all the answers, but I know some of them.

I know that my Belgian grandparents Antoine and Alice both spoke fluent English to my mother because they both had stayed in England during World War I. Recent research has shocked me that 250,000 Belgian refugees came to the UK during that war, the largest immigrant influx in UK history with 16,000 arriving in Folkestone on 14th October 1914. They also landed at other Kent ports, including Dover and Margate, but also at Tilbury, Hull, Grimsby and Harwich. Purpose-built Belgian villages sprang up, but the majority were housed across the UK.

After the war, the government policy was to get the soldiers back and the Belgian refugees out. They were encouraged to go home with employment contracts terminated and even given free one-way boat tickets. The Belgian government also encouraged the refugees to come home. Within 12 months of November 1918, 90% had returned home. My Belgian grandparents were amongst that 225,000 that returned home.

My father was born in Eckeren outside of Antwerp in June 1925, like me the middle of three brothers. His elder brother Anthony (Antoine anglicised) was highly active in the resistance opposing the German occupation of Belgium in the Second World War. He went on the run and tried to escape to Switzerland, but I gather was shot by the Germans near the border. My father never got on well with his younger brother, my Uncle Paul, and hinted at family business problems with my grandfather's wine and beer retail business, but there were also darker hints about my uncle's death. It was the first time I ever heard of a resistance cell where within the resistance you only know a limited number of members and if someone in the cell is betrayed, suspicion falls on remaining members of the cell. The smaller the number for a resistance cell, the fewer participants can be betrayed and the fewer suspects, so if one member is arrested the second member knows it is not him and that means suspicion falls on the remaining cell members. My Uncle Anthony was in a small resistance cell, so my father was always a little suspicious of my Uncle Paul's role in his betrayal.

Years later, one of our vets was from Antwerp and she rang all the Paul Sauvages in the directory and was sure she spoke to my Uncle Paul or a near relative, but the phone was put down. As a child I remember my elder brother and father going to Antwerp as my grandmother Alice was ill and I remember my uncle coming to see us once, but I think the reconciliation was short-lived.

I always thought my maternal grandmother, whose maiden name was Maud Daw, came from Canterbury. I was shocked recently to discover that she was born in 1888 in Fleet, Hampshire, the same place as my wife. To jump forward several years, I was skiing with a friend Bruce, who was MD of a veterinary drug company at the time, when he told me his father was a GP in Fleet. Much to my surprise, I found out from my mother-in-law that, yes, that same Dr Robinson delivered my wife Sandra.

Her husband William Wood had served in the trenches in the first war. He stayed with us for a while in the 60s and always seemed a nice person to me although upset my mother occasionally and never got on with his estranged wife. My mother was born in June 1912 in England before World War I but brought up in India where my grandfather was the kennel man for the Maharaja of Jind. My aunt was born in India. The city of Jind is north-west of New Delhi.

One day when my mother was about 11 years-old, she was playing in a village clearing when out of the jungle a glassy-eyed medium-sized mongrel dog emerged. The dog was wobbly and salivating and attacked an old rubber tyre the kids used to play with. My mother immediately yelled at the other kids that the dog had rabies. Rabies is a zoonosis, a disease that spreads from animals to man usually via bites as saliva is rich in the virus and over-salivation is a common symptom, as are behavioural changes. These are usually aggressive behaviour but occasionally not, so-called dumb rabies. It is caused by a virus that attacks the nervous system. It can now be prevented by vaccination of both humans and animals and has allowed the recent Pet Passport system.

All the kids scattered and thanks to her nobody got bitten but as she was sprinting down a little narrow pathway within close range of the clearing she tripped and fell flat on her face. With blood and tears streaming down her face, fearing the dog was not far behind, she jumped straight up and sprinted home. The local doctor said she had severe nose and facial fractures and had to go by train to a hospital. She told me of the long painful overnight train journey to Delhi for hospitalisation and treatment.

Because of the rising Indian Independence movement, it was becoming increasingly unsafe for an English family in India and after several threats and an increasingly unhappy marriage between my grandparents, they decided to leave and get back to England. The breaking family were certainly back in England by the beginning of the war in 1939 and my English grandfather and grandmother had gone their separate ways. There was an elder brother also called Will

Wood and he became a policeman in Colchester, and everyone called him "Tim" as in Timber Wood. He had a daughter, a cousin I met a couple of times when we were kids and I met Tim. The two families were not close although I knew my mother was very fond of Tim.

When war broke out, my mother and my aunt were living with my grandmother somewhere near Knights Hill, not far from Crystal Palace. The two sisters volunteered for the London Auxiliary Ambulance Service (LAAS) which was set up on the outbreak of war. The stations were manned by 80 volunteers for 24 hours a day. The drivers were all women, and the stretcher bearers were men. Many of the vehicles were donated and converted to ambulances with wire-mesh solid stretchers: the type of stretcher I remember seeing as a boy joined end to end to make fencing on top of low walls around council flats. They were issued Civil Defence uniforms and badges in 1941 and I have pictures of my mother and aunt wearing them. There is also an undated press cutting of a children's party held by her LAAS branch one Saturday morning in those uniforms, so obviously taken before the main children's evacuations from London during the Blitz of 1940-42.

One other thing I know is that my mother was in the Rose and Crown pub at Crown Point, Knights Hill, when it was bombed. I am not sure of the date, but the attack was recorded in the Aggregate night-time Bomb Census 7/10/40 -6/6/41. My mother described a beam trapping her legs and several fatalities including the landlord found dead in his bath in the nearby Crown Lane.

I know she then drove lorries for the NAAFI (Navy Army Air Force Institute) including into liberated Belgium and ended up spending some time in the NAAFI run "21 Club" where she met my father.

He had started work in several of the large hotels in occupied Antwerp from 1940 including the Hotel Metropole and after playing a run-on part in the liberation of Antwerp ended up in the 21 Club as a waiter.

There are some wedding pictures in a park in Antwerp taken in July 1946. My brother was born back in England in March 1947. My father was on his death bed when he told me the story of his role in the liberation of Antwerp. I had asked him why he was so apolitical and never voted. He said that he was brought up in an era where men like Adolf Hitler said they would build roads and built them, said they would deal with unemployment and did so, then he realised all the political promises led to war. He then mentioned the liberation of Belgium, saying there were all the Belgian politicians sitting in London broadcasting on Free Belgian Radio encouraging Belgians to fight and liberate the homeland. He and two friends were enthusiastic enough to get weapons from resistance contacts and charge across a bridge to dislodge the Germans during the liberation of Antwerp. The friend on his left was shot dead, the friend on his right was wounded and my father had bullet holes in his trousers.

"What made me lose all faith in politicians after that was," he said, "my friend's family had to pay for his funeral and his wounded friend got a hospital bill." I asked why and he said because they were not "Officially Recognised Freedom Fighters" and "you ask why I never vote?" He felt well enough to laugh when I asked, "Did the government pay for your trousers?" In the same conversation he told me how this unrecognised status helped him when he was trying to get British nationalisation just as the Congo war started; he was called back to Belgium for National Service, destined for what looked like a bloody war of Independence in the Congo. He was asked if he had any weapon training or experience and he replied he had not, only catering training, hoping his officially unrecognised fighter status still stood. Nobody ever found a war record and he spent the time in Belgium sorting catering supplies for the distant army. My father's National Service was soon over and he was back in England, finally obtaining British nationality in 1959.

5

THE RVC

Many people get confused when talking of the Royal Veterinary College (RVC) and the Royal College of Veterinary Surgeons (RCVS)

The RVC is the veterinary college based in Royal College Street, Camden Town, London, with a field station at Potters Bar in Hertfordshire. It is one of the universities in the UK where veterinary degrees are offered. The job title is abbreviated colloquially in Britain to vets and in the USA we are known as veterinarians.

The Royal College of Veterinary Surgeons is the governing body of all qualified UK vets. There is inevitable confusion when people talk of the Royal College, but they usually mean the RCVS and to be a practising vet in the UK you need to be a member of the RCVS and have the title MRCVS. Because they are surgeons, vets have been traditionally addressed as Mr, Mrs or Miss but not Doctor, although this is changing with most vets elsewhere in the world called Doctor.

So, in September 1968 I attended the RVC as a student for the first time but here is the litmus test: I was a member of the RVC but not a member of the RCVS. I was awarded the MRCVS on 10th April 1973, almost five years later because of graduating from the RVC.

Anyway, in September 1968 within a month of my A level results and less than a month after my acceptance, here I was in Camden Town after an induction day at the RVC.

We ended the day at a drinks reception in the same hall with the picture of George III looking down on me as I nervously chatted with my fellow freshers and several lecturers and the Principal in the same room. I remember a few of the characters that I would come to know very well over the next few years. Professor Hancock, Head of Anatomy; Mr Vaughan, an orthopaedic surgeon; Mr Churchill-Frost, another surgeon; Miss Jenny Poland, a pathologist; a lovely tall bald gentleman called Mr Greatorex but even then I was told his name was Johnny G – probably by the student assigned to show us around.

The sherry was flowing so my lack of confidence was dampened, and I joined the circle around him as one of the fresher ladies, obviously very horsey, asked him why horses get colic so frequently. I had no idea what they were talking about except I knew babies got colic and guessed it was a sort of belly ache.

One thing I learned very quickly that evening was to shut up and listen or ask a sensible question. Johnny G answered her with the comment that given how complicated a horse's digestive system was, he was surprised they did not get colic more often. I knew nothing about a horse gut, but the sherry talked, and I asked, "Was a horse's gut system like a rabbit's?" My horsey year-mate's jaw dropped at the thought of comparing her beloved horses with a rabbit and I went red with embarrassment, feeling my first day of vet college was not going well. Johnny G came to my rescue with the comment, "Exactly like a rabbit: a single stomach, a great big large intestine and a massive caecum." My confidence grew and I even went to the pub, "The Parrs Head" in Camden Town, with my new-found friends before getting on the tube home.

The rest of the term it was down to study at Camden Town, working on the so-called pre-clinical subjects of anatomy, physiology, biochemistry, physical chemistry, genetics and pharmacology with Fridays at Potters Bar doing animal husbandry – and just the odd visit for me to the college bar or the Parrs Head.

I joined the college football team, but my ability had not suddenly improved. This was a time long before substitutes so I was asked to referee. I enjoyed it and went on a referee course with another member of the team who was also in my year. Within three months we were qualified as FA approved referees. Dave was a good striker so he went back to playing and I refereed. At the end of the first match one my ex-teammates said, "You were a rubbish player and a rubbish ref, now you are a rubbish qualified ref, so I must not complain."

I remember two matches clearly, one against the Royal College of Music. They were a team the RVC usually beat but their goalkeeper this game pulled off a stunning series of saves, including a point-blank shot from Dave. This last shot bent his fingers right back and when I congratulated him on the way he was playing he told me he was a pianist and must not injure his hands. Within minutes he let in three goals and was reluctant to shake hands with anyone after the game.

The other memorable event was when the centre half, also called Dave, rolled off the back of the opposing centre forward and we all heard a loud crack like a twig snapping and he said he had fractured his collar bone. I pressed at the site and felt the characteristic crepitus of a fracture. I said, "Yes, Dave, you have a fracture, I can feel crepitus." Another ten members of the vet student team came up and pressed at the injury saying, "Yes, that's crepitus." At which point Wally the groundsman took Dave to casualty. When I saw Dave years later at a vet conference in Jerusalem, he mentioned how our medical curiosity outweighed our sympathies whilst he suffered.

I carried on refereeing matches not only for the college but throughout London until I qualified, and got to a fairly high level running a line for the level below the Football League by the time I qualified as a vet.

The year went well and before we knew it, it was time for exams. The first-year examination in June was not a problem as I had had to work so hard for A levels I was in the swing of studying. Sadly, some of my year did not fare so well with some failing one or two exams and having to re-sit after the summer break. The biggest causes of the failures I think was the attraction of bridge, chess, and the fact that two or three spent the whole of first year lectures reading the "Lord of the Rings". The bright lights of London must also share some of the blame.

About eleven of these very bright students ended up being dumped out of the course after failing the resits in September. Another major factor was that some of them thought as they had breezed through O levels and cruised through A levels that they could do the same at first year vet school with the same work rate. I had always struggled academically but unlike my sports playing I did not take my eye off the ball. Unlike the re-sit group, I enjoyed my summer with a camping trip to Jersey with some friends I had known since primary school, Colin and Martin.

I also continued my long-term student job that I had been doing for several years in Streatham Bingo Hall. I had worked in the Prize Bingo area at the back of the stage where during breaks from the cash bingo a mini prize bingo unit was set up. My job entailed all roles from cashier to calling the numbers including all the rhymes and reminders such as "The next number out is number one on its own, number one".

The prize bingo ran between the two sessions of cash bingo and during the interval twice a day, afternoon and evening, seven days a week so there were plenty of breaks for studying for my A levels and then my vet studies. The bingo hall manager went to the Abbey Road Offices in early September 1969 looking for sponsorship for the English Apple Week promotion being run nationally; he obtained two signed copies of the Beatles album "Abbey Road". They were signed across the zebra crossing below each of the four Beatles.

One was given away as a prize, the other signed cover was put in the "shop window" and given to me when the window display was taken down in late 1969 when I did my last student spell there over the Christmas and New Year of 1969-70. I added my shop-purchased LP to the signed cover and kept it in my possession along with several other LPs also given to me at the time obtained from the same trip to Abbey Road Offices. I have kept them ever since and always believed them to be genuine signatures until I took them to see Stephen Maycock, Bonhams Entertainment Consultant, last year. He accepted the provenance but whilst looking at the signed Abbey Road cover told me many people including family members signed autographs on behalf of members of the band.

Neil Aspinall, the road manager and later Apple manager, was a prolific signer and members of the band occasionally signed for each other. Neil Aspinall even signed the band's equity applications and cards to allow them to act in the two Beatles films. Stephen's opinion was that all four signatures were not by the band, although the George Harrison signature was good, but the other signatures encouraged his opinion that this too was signed by another. He stated that the original autographs of the band members changed with time except Ringo's, which is still terribly like those signed in the 1960s. He commented that the album is 50 years old this year (2019), so the value is about £20, the same as any other copy except this one has been misleadingly defaced.

There was never any intention to defraud by these false signings but simply to satisfy public demand without further pressure on the band members. The signed cover would have been extremely valuable if genuine, but it will always be a special reminder to me of that job which I had to give up as from then on my student holidays would be full with so-called "Seeing Practice". This meant spending twenty-six weeks in a veterinary practice between college terms from then on until I qualified, plus two weeks to be spent on a farm the following summer as part of the animal husbandry course.

6

FIRST YEAR BVETMED

The end of my second year at the RVC meant passing a formal pre-clinical examination in all the subjects I previously listed plus histology, the study of cells and tissues. These were the First BVetMed exams; with animal husbandry, which comprised part of the formal second BVetMed examination, in March of the third year.

As I said, I was lucky enough to do O level in anatomy and physiology, so I understood the basics of both these subjects, but the depth was tremendous and involved a lot of hard work. Our first term of first year anatomy was a very well taught course on the domestic cat, starting with the skeleton then covering digestive, reproductive, respiratory, circulatory, and skin systems. In the following terms we had to spend a term each on dog, cow and horse anatomy. Each of these involved dissections of these different species and the smell of the preservative formalin was familiar from A level zoology but scaled up to eye watering proportions.

The cattle dissection involved a frame suspending the carcass in a big Victorian lecture theatre where we sat around the professor and his assistant as they dissected with help from us. The assistant was a charming, helpful man who was slightly older than us and in polio leg irons to help him walk and I suspect from his limited upper body movement he also had a back support, but he was as strong as the ox he was dissecting, and I was so grateful I had avoided this terrible disease and been vaccinated with my sugar lump.

The next term the process was repeated with a horse suspended in the frame as we learnt about the horse's nervous system, helped by the professor's assistant suspended in his frame from the damage done to his nervous system by a terrible virus. The professor was full of great stories and while talking about the blood vessels that run inside the neck vertebra of a horse, he told us that rabbits had the same channel for an artery in their neck vertebra and whilst having a rabbit casserole in a restaurant in Camden Town during the war he pulled a neck bone out of his so-called rabbit stew and identified the bone from the fact it did not have the canal as belonging to one of the few species that did not – a guinea pig.

In the anatomy museum at the college was the skeleton of the famous horse Eclipse: he is known as the grandfather of modern racing and I spent hours in front of that skeleton learning the bones and then mentally putting flesh on those bones in the form of tendons, ligaments nerves muscles and then filling him with heart, lungs, liver, and that complex digestive system and finally skin before going back to the bare bones. He is now in the building named after him in the college in Hertfordshire.

Knowing the casualty rate from the first-year exam, everyone took the end-of-year exam seriously and I was often not alone staring at Eclipse with the professor's notes in hand. I always believed the hardest thing about vet college was getting admitted; staying there was tough work but now the odds were in my favour if I studied hard.

After the second-year exams the results were quickly published, with a few more re-sits and two forced to leave. It was time to really focus on animal husbandry. The next step was the farm practice and a written project about the farm. I was invited to Devon to stay with a friend in my year, Paul, while we both worked at a farm in the north of the county near Bideford. It was a mixed arable livestock farm with sheep and North Devon cattle. I had no farming background and had to learn fast how to feed the yarded cattle, a beef breed, respect the bull and check the sheep.

The farmer and his family were exceedingly kind to Paul and me but one of the aspects that needed discussion in the written project was the economics of the farm. It is difficult to talk to anyone about their income and neither Paul nor I could see a way forward. It was almost our last day on the farm when I got the farmer alone on a tractor and knew it was now or never. Once I worked up the courage, I asked which was the best part of the enterprise economically: the cattle, the sheep or the arable. He replied without hesitation, the cattle, and went into detail.

Since North Devons are a beef breed for meat, the flock of sheep just helped clear up the grazing land and the lamb sales did not add much to the family income. The arable crops, mainly barley, were used to feed the yarded cattle on a three-year system when the bullocks were ready for slaughter. He said the profits were very variable, but the farm was not mortgaged, and he owned the freehold. In a good year he could buy new equipment and in a bad year he could not. I think he found it helpful to talk to a relative stranger about his financial problems. Paul was shocked when later that night I told him all the last details we needed for our projects.

7

SNOW ANGELS

The third year was devoted to more animal husbandry and a new group of subjects. Pathology, the study of disease; parasitology, the study of parasitic animals such as worms, fleas, lice, etc.; bacteriology, the study of bacteria; and virology, the study of viruses. Imagine how frustrating I find it when I read the scientific correspondents of eminent newspapers talking of "bugs" when they mean viruses, or "germs" when they mean bacteria – or often they are unsure what they do mean.

After passing the animal husbandry project it was the end of Easter term 1971 and we were terribly busy learning the academic part of the course and planning our extra-mural practice.

The first extra-mural work was to support our pathology training, so I went for two weeks before Easter to a Veterinary Investigation (VI) Centre at Worcester; the work was remarkably interesting with many poultry, cattle and sheep post-mortem investigations and laboratory testing of the samples taken. I had driven to Worcester in a little Hillman Imp that I had had for a few years. It was a typical student's car, always breaking down, but it was not a mechanical failure that caused a problem on the way home from Worcester. It was a blizzard.

The snow started to fall when I left about 3.30 that Friday afternoon and snow and ice was quickly making the roads very slippery and treacherous. I eventually got stuck trying to get up a hill and the car would just slide to the bottom of the hill again. After about my third attempt to get up the hill I had slid into the near-side kerb, so I jumped out of the car to check my rear tyre against the kerb. It was outside a large Victorian style house with a large drive and I could hear children shouting and playing in the snow. It is all right for you I thought as I jumped into the car and tried to slalom up the hill again. I had only got about 10 yards up this time when the car stopped, wheels racing, and started sliding back down the hill.

"We will push you," shouted a young voice behind me and suddenly I saw in my rear-view mirror little hands appearing on my rear windscreen as the car was pushed. We made it up the hill easily thanks to the screaming and cheering children all pushing, some of them pushing from the sides but most from the back. At the top of the hill with the car on level ground I got out to thank the children who had helped me, especially when adults had rushed by with their own pedestrian problems of getting home in a snowstorm. I was shocked to see each child who had pushed me had horrible arm deformities with little malformed hands appearing to come straight from their torsos. There were about a dozen of them, the eldest was about eleven, but some were several years younger. The Victorian house must have been a home for the children of Thalidomide.

They seemed such jolly happy kids in each other's company with the most positive attitude. I profusely thanked them with tears in my eyes, but they just ran down the hill laughing to resume their game in the garden or perhaps wait for another car to get stuck.

They were my Snow Angels and they got me home safely. I had learnt many new words in my pathology classes that year and "iatrogenic" was one of them: it means, broadly, illness caused by medical examination or treatment but more specifically and usually drug-induced illness. Thalidomide was used in pregnant women throughout the world between 1957 and 1962 for various problems in pregnancy; when the connection was finally made that it caused many deformities in the developing foetus, including limb deformities, it was withdrawn in 1961. My little Snow Angels had literally been dealt a terrible hand in life, but they seemed to be determined to make the most of it.

It is a sad statistic world-wide that fewer than 3,000 are still alive. Anyone who argues against animal experimentation must confront the fact that had Thalidomide been trialled on pregnant monkeys the drug would not have been released and 10,000 deformed babies would not have been born. I had just had a tough term with animal death and post-mortem change, but those kids taught me how special human life was and animal life, whilst particularly important, was not in the same category. At the VI Lab they often encouraged vets to send in live chickens from a diseased flock so these birds could be sacrificed, and the illness more efficiently investigated. This is a tough line to take to kill animals for the greater human or animal good, but veganism is the only alternative which, if taken to its logical conclusion, means fewer animals in the world, not more.

8

2ND YEAR BVETMED

We were due to sit the second BVetMed exams comprising of pathology, including parasitology, etc., and animal husbandry and veterinary hygiene which also included meat Inspection the following March, 1972, so I had two years from the Easter Veterinary Investigation Centre to complete my seeing practice time. I calculated I could just fit this in all the various holiday times and would have time to drive into Europe that summer camping with Ian, a friend from college. I made it to Dubrovnik and back with one major breakdown, a clutch replacement at Split.

The drive to Yugoslavia, as it was known then, was exciting and involved going across Germany, over the Austrian Alps and into northern Italy, then over the border into Yugoslavia. My main memory in Germany was stopping for a few days in the Black Forest town of Baden Baden and enjoying the beer kellers. I was shocked when swimming at a local pool how many of the middle-aged population had lost limbs in the war. I found the people very friendly but was surprised on the campsite how they laughed, albeit in a pleasant manner, at our primitive tents and primus stoves which were pump-up stoves using smelly blue methylated spirit. They all seemed to have small blue cylinder-driven gas lights and cookers and were obviously worried about the mad English setting light to the campsite with our little ancient stoves.

We finally got to Yugoslavia which is now divided into modern Croatia, Serbia, Montenegro, Kosovo, and Bosnia and Herzegovina. It was led at the time by independent Communist Tito. During our visit there we detected none of the internal religious or nationalist movements that were to tear the country apart with civil war from 1989. The only detectable animosity was towards the Germans: all the locals in our campsites on the coast trip south from Split to Dubrovnik seemed to be against them and welcomed the British with open arms.

When the car broke down there were many communication difficulties with the mechanic repairing it and language was one. He spoke no English but good German, so we had to get an English-speaking German who had also broken down to translate for us. The problem was he innately hated the poor German and wanted to help us while very reluctant to repair the German's engine. By the end of the week, he had repaired my estate car's clutch and the German's was next if and when the part he needed arrived from Belgrade. The history of the German invasion and occupation of 1941 was not easily forgotten and certainly not forgiven.

Because of the delay caused by the breakdown we decided to drive up the last bit of the coast road to Dubrovnik overnight, sharing the driving. During daylight, the views from the road winding by the sea were fantastic; at some stages the road was on the cliff top high above the sea with a completely unprotected drop off to the right into the sea far below. The route south was particularly interesting because we were driving on the right with right-hand drive and oncoming traffic including big trucks appearing round a bend coming straight at us with only the cliff edge on our right.

Daylight was scary enough, but night-time was certainly interesting. On one of my shifts that night at about 2am I was stuck behind one of the large dumper-style trucks heading towards the south like us. There was no way we could pass him but a good job we did not. I woke Ian and shouted, "Hey look at this truck," as he started weaving on the road about 500 yards above the rocky moonlit coastline, "I think the driver in front is falling asleep." The lorry weaved again and a wheel nearly went over the edge. I flashed my lights and intermittently sounded the horn, by which time the lorry was over to the left in danger of oncoming traffic or crashing into the cliff wall on our left. I had to back off in case he crashed but kept honking the horn and flashing the headlights. Suddenly the lorry straightened as the driver awoke. Shortly there was a lay-by to the left, and he pulled into it, waving his thanks as we drove by.

We went on to the amazing walled city of Dubrovnik and found a campsite just outside. The idyllic stay was marred only by Ian getting a severe bout of gastro-enteritis and being confined to the campsite, or more specifically the campsite toilet block, for two days.

As a result of organising the trip to Yugoslavia that summer, I was asked on my return to college the next term to apply to go on the East African Research Trip. I had not applied as I felt I would be short of my 26 weeks seeing practice if I spent the following summer in Africa, but the team leader Bob persuaded me to apply and I was accepted onto the team. This meant that I would now have to spend all my non-term time in a foster practice and I would have to give up any idea of supplementing my grant with student holiday work between then and qualification.

The research project in Africa was a tradition at the RVC with a team going out and carrying out some useful veterinary work for one of the East African countries, usually Kenya. My trip should involve a trip to Uganda where we would test for the presence of brucellosis, a bacterial cause of abortion in cattle but also a zoonosis (disease spread from animals to humans) causing Undulant Fever in people, as well as monitoring the worm and fluke parasite status of the country's cattle. We would also TB test the cattle – another zoonosis.

The whole trip required raising funds and my responsibility was to get sponsorship from companies that had previously helped us. By now I had moved out from my parents and was in a flat in Stamford Hill with three other students from my year. I spent my evenings studying or typing on an old typewriter letters to potential sponsors: slowly and painfully my typing speeded up. I say I was in the flat with three guys from my year: one of them had decided to stay pre-clinical for a year and do a BSc, so I remember Dickey talking of a reproductive hormone I had never heard of called prostaglandin. Within five years this drug revolutionised cattle fertility treatment with the trade name "Estrumate", just showing how quickly medicine can move forward on occasions.

One of my main problems that year was financial. The amount of grant given to me by my local council was meant to be subsidised by my parents, but I never got the parental contribution from my father. I had not expected him to pay when I lived at home but when I moved out he still did not pay it and I had no holiday time to earn money. I was not the only poor student, as many had trouble eking out their grant. The amount the council paid was calculated according to parental earnings, so the more a family earned the smaller the grant and the greater the parental contribution.

Dickey had no grant that year as he was doing the BSc. The net result was that we were broke and, like so many students before us and after, spent too much on beer at the pub – my other flatmates, Neil and Mike, more so than the average. They were always in the pub. The current government student loan system is the cause of a lot of complaint, but I think it is a fair system and students will always be hard up no matter what the financial system they study in. We did have one great advantage over present students in that we did not have to pay the college fees – they were also paid by our local authorities.

That year we were particularly broke, and I remember Neil bringing back at the beginning of term a bag of pig feed quality potatoes from Somerset which we paid him for and buying a dozen cracked eggs a week from the college farm as we were there once a week. It was no surprise that we regularly went home for weekends. We got fed and our washing done, and Neil stacked up our pig feed potatoes. Regarding the washing, years later one of our bachelor vets went one step further: on his weekends off he rattled round the motorway from Kent to Chelmsford to see his family not only with his dirty washing but with a box full of his washing-up from the last few weeks working in the practice to not only make use of his family washing machine but the family dishwasher as well.

To raise funds for the East African Research Team we organised an "Animal Scramble". Each year of the RVC had to build itself a large, mobile model animal which was to be pushed/pulled to the Agricultural College in Wye in Kent seventy miles away, which was the most distant college of London University.

It was proposed that we set off in the early hours of 29th November. I cannot remember all the different animals, there was certainly a zebra and a giraffe, but they were all spectacular and some very well designed, light and could be towed by a cycle. The exception was the first year's choice. They decided to papier-mâché up the jumping horse from the college gym as a rhinoceros. They ended up with a great heavy cumbersome beast but an equally attractive one. We all set off before first light with several support cars, and our team and most of the others covered 40 miles to just south-west of Maidstone by about 9am, when we were not meant to be in the designated pub, The Tickled Trout, at West Farleigh in Kent, until lunchtime. The frequent changes of pushers, pullers and cyclists from the back-up cars helped us all make excellent time; sadly, I remember the landlord did not open for us or even greet us out of his window. We also raced by another pub, The Battle of Britain, but it was still too early for a drink there as well. We were so ahead of schedule. Years later my parents owned a bungalow almost opposite this pub but I never did get in there. Because of the fitness of most of the students, all the animals except one were at Wye by lunchtime.

The celebratory party was well under way when the exhausted first years arrived about 9pm pushing just a piece of gym equipment. The animal had disintegrated, and it took them until the end of term to get it in a van back to Camden Town. All the years and the staff raised several hundreds of pounds in sponsorship, so the Animal Scramble was a great success. Wye College sadly closed in 2005.

At the end of each term, we were out in practice ticking off our twenty-six weeks and so much depended on the practice that accepted you as a student. More of that later as the Second BVetMed exams loomed in March 1972.

The examinations were both written and oral. After a weekend of swatting, the exam paper on veterinary pathology was in front of us at 10am. We had three hours to answer six questions on virology, bacteriology and parasitology. That afternoon from 2.30, the same format on pathology but this time more focused on diseases such as anaemia and chronic renal disease of dogs and vitamin deficiencies. The following day, the same format for hygiene and husbandry and by 5.30pm that day my head was spinning. If I seem to remember a lot of detail it is because where possible I have always kept exam papers. To me the oral part of the examination process was straightforward after the difficult written papers.

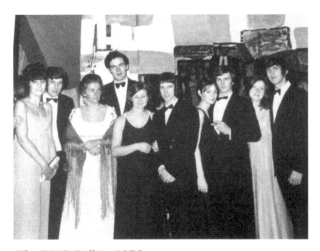

The RVC Ball in 1972

9

SEEING PRACTICE

I first saw practice for two weeks in Streatham at a dog and cat practice. Dick Vonesch was a talented surgeon able to carry out intricate spinal surgery, including a fracture of the odontoid peg in a miniature poodle. The dog was presented to him on my first morning surgery having been dropped on its head after jumping out of its owner's arms; he was screaming with pain on presentation and quickly needed sedation, then a general anaesthetic and the x-ray clearly showed separation due to a fracture of the odontoid peg, a small tooth-like protrusion of the axis bone, the second cervical (neck) vertebra which supports the atlas, the first neck vertebra.

It is amazing that having seen this one I have not seen another case since and that was 50 years ago. Dick stabilised the atlas to the axis with wire on each side of the axis allowing the little peg to heal. From the day of surgery, the dog showed no more neck pain. Dick was the vet for Battersea Dogs Home where he did regular work for them as at the time they did not have their own vet. The fact it was 50 years ago was further demonstrated because when we went there, as well as doing a clinic checking several dogs, he showed me the electrocutor. This was used to euthanase unwanted dogs that were usually sick, often showing signs of distemper. Everyone at Battersea, including Dick, reassured me how humane this was. I was unsure of the reasoning for this: it just seemed more convenient than the traditional intravenous drug overdose using barbiturate. Fortunately, I did not see this horror machine in action, but I saw the tray ready to be filled with water that the dog stood in and the clips attached at various points on the body before a high current passed through. It seems that my feelings on this are now accepted and it is many years since Battersea used this barbaric piece of equipment.

I next saw practice in a mixed practice seeing horses, cattle, sheep as well as dogs and cats in Oxted, Kent. The vets and staff there were lovely, but an unpleasant head nurse did not make for a good learning experience. The first day I got taken out by the senior partner and thoroughly investigated some lame horses. One was hopping lame until some pus was cut out from the sole of its front hoof, the second was more complicated and would probably need x-rays later in the week if it did not settle with pain killers. The next day I was shepherded away from the horse visits and made to just sit around, not being allowed into the operating theatre. I sat all morning reading textbooks from the practice library.

On the Wednesday, the third day of my week in Oxted, I managed to chat to the vet surgeon who did all the ops in theatre and although she invited me into theatre to scrub up and join in, I was quickly shooed away by the senior nurse again. On Thursday, the lame horse came in for x-ray and I hoped to witness the procedure but was sent on a house call with one of the vets to vaccinate a cat against a disease known as panleucopaenia, a virus of the parvovirus family. More of that disease later. By the time I got back, as cats always hide on house calls, it was too late to see the x-ray procedure and had to just look at the textbooks again. It was by the Thursday evening surgery that I found out the head nurse was a Crystal Palace fan, a team I had supported since I was a boy. I asked her if she was going to the match on Saturday and she replied she was but if you think this story has a happy ending, think again, as the next day I was briefly allowed into theatre to watch a bitch spay from a distance before being ushered out to the books.

There was no routine operating on a Saturday but there was a different atmosphere in the practice that morning without the nurse's presence and I saw some interesting cases while she went to football.

My week in Oxted was over and I was determined to find a more suitable practice before Christmas, which was only a week or so away.

We were living in Beckenham then and my father was commuting to his job as the banqueting manager of the Great Danes Hotel just outside Maidstone. He suggested I look at the market town of Kent for a suitable practice. It had to be a mixed practice and he brought me a local directory from work. Finding Crowhurst and Partners in the *Yellow Pages*, the following Monday morning I gave them a ring. An extremely helpful telephone receptionist answered my call. I told them I was a vet student and she put me through to one of the vets. He told me his name was John Crossley. "We haven't got a student with us at the moment, why not come down this afternoon at 2.30," he said.

I grabbed my white coat and Wellington boots and set off for Maidstone in my car, allowing plenty of time, and got a bit lost in the town with its one-way system looking for Museum Street. By the Carriage Museum was a map so I parked and looked up Museum Street and saw it was nowhere near that museum but at the junction of Earl Street. I parked in the practice yard and was quickly told by one of the nurses that I was in Mr Crowhurst's parking spot. Here we go again, I thought, but once my car was moved everyone was pleasant and I was taken into the office and met JC. He was a charming man who after a smiley greeting said, "Get your boots, we are off."

What a great day I had. We saw a lame horse and he asked me the likely cause of sudden lameness. "Pus in the foot," I said hopefully.

"Good chance; common things occur commonly," JC replied. We arrived at the stable and jumped out of the car. "This is John our student," he introduced me to the head-scarfed, beautifully spoken client. "I think she has pulled her near shoulder," she said as we walked across the stable yard. After trotting her, JC asked me which side her head nodded when placing her foot. "Left," I said. "Yes," said JC, "she nods on her near side."

The client repeated her diagnosis about the mare's near shoulder. JC, to humour the client, went to the left shoulder and ran the palm of his hands over the area. "They nod on the sound side," he whispered to me as he walked round the head end of the horse and ran the palm of his hand over the right/off shoulder and down the leg, feeling the hoof. "That's hot," as he leaned against the horse and lifted her leg. With his hoof knife, a strange knife with a hooked blade at the end, he pared at the horse's sole, tapping around the sole with the handle of the knife. He pared the V-shaped frog, the spongy tissue that led to the heel, and returned to tapping the sole. It was obvious the lovely hunter mare was more uncomfortable when he tapped the inner part of the sole to the left of the frog at 9 o'clock on the clock face if the frog was 6 o'clock, and was unmoved by tapping at 3 o'clock. He started to pare deeply where the flinching was most and suddenly a jet of muck leaked out. She indeed had pus in the foot and seemed mightily relieved to have it released. Once he had given an injection of antibiotics and anti-tetanus, he advised a warm compress on the foot and said we would come back the next day and repeat the antibiotic injection and see how she was.

"Common things occur commonly," he said again as we sped off in his car. "Where now?" I asked but did not get a reply until we arrived at one of the least smelly pig farms I had been to up to that point. We jumped out and I was handed several metal containers of glass syringes and needles and a dark treacly drug bottle. We put on our wellies and coats and jumped into a pigsty full of squealing juvenile pigs. The weaners were given 2ml each of the liquid and lifted into a neighbouring pen. Originally, I held them and JC injected into the rear leg just above the hock. "Which muscle?" asked JC. "Gastrocnemius," was my reply.

"Good man," he said, as he handed me the syringe. I then injected my first live animals; filling the syringe with the iron supplement to prevent anaemia was harder than injecting it. The syringe disconnected from the needle when I was injecting once, and the thick liquid went everywhere. JC laughed even though some went on his face as he was holding the piglet upside down. "Good job the farmer didn't see that. By the way, where is the farmer?" I said with embarrassment. "He did see it," JC replied, "This is my pig farm."

He then drove me back to the practice, explaining that we had gone to the horse first as horses hate the smell of pigs.

The next day I went back to the lame mare and JC told me to take the poultice off and explore the foot; I further explored the little carved pit, and no more pus came out.

I then was asked to inject the mare with her antibiotics. The technique was as I had seen the day before. Sterilise the neck skin with a cotton wool swab, then tap the horse's neck, ending with a little series of slaps and on the last slap stick in the needle; if no blood, connect the syringe and draw back on the plunger again once to make sure not in a blood vessel. Then inject, making sure syringe, needle and horse stay in alignment if any movement by the horse.

It worked well and the client seemed happy to let me do what JC instructed but there was a relief on both mine and the client's face when the injection went well, and JC gave her a reassuring look. It was very empowering to be trusted.

JC never told me where we were going, and he pulled in the driveway of a lovely Kentish farmhouse at Hunton near Yalding and I asked if we were seeing a horse. "Yes," he replied as we walked to the stable and looked at a beautiful bay hunter gelding leaning over the stable door. I offered to get a head collar, but he said do not worry, when a lady came out of the house yelling that he was late. He introduced me to his wife, Mrs C, whose bark was loud, but she did not bite. She greeted me like a long-lost nephew and ushered me into the lovely hall of the house with its beams and inglenooks through to the kitchen where the table was laid up for lunch.

The phone has not stopped, she shouted to JC from the other end of the kitchen. A neighbour has rung to say her cat has chewed through the wires of the Christmas lights. JC asked what she had said. "I'm not a vet," she screamed. "I told her it was a bit shocked and to keep it warm until you can ring back." We all then laughed at her joke while JC rang the neighbour and said we would drop in and see the cat in an hour as it seemed fine. After a tremendous three-course lunch of soup, cold meat, salad and potatoes and traditional spotted dick and custard pudding, I could see where JC got his paunch from.

We then went next door to see the cat. It was of course nowhere to be seen but was eventually found under a bed. It was a little 12-week-old kitten and on examination was depressed with a red burn mark across the hard palate. JC gave it an under the skin (subcutaneous – SC) injection in the scruff of the neck as opposed to in the muscle (IM). Those who have needle phobia, look away now! He showed me how to make a pyramid-shaped tent out of the scruff of the neck using finger and thumb, then inject at the bottom of the pyramid without putting the needle in, then out of the tent. Once in, inject after withdrawing on the plunger a little to make sure no blood. The neighbour then asked what about her light, especially her Christmas tree lights in the lounge? It was an old property like JC's, and I found the fuse box and luckily found some fuse wire on the box. I repaired the old fuse and the lights all worked: good job it was low ampage wire – that had saved the kitten from a fatal electric shock. "I trust you are not charging for a visit as you are just next door," said the neighbour. JC laughed and said we were not charging for repairing the fuse and we left.

I had a couple of days off for Christmas, but I was looking forward to seeing practice between Christmas and New Year in the knowledge I had found the perfect foster practice.

JC had the time between Christmas and New Year off, so I went on several cattle calls with a recent graduate called Stuart. The calls including a great big Friesian cow with milk fever, a typical case just gone down after calving at a local farm outside of Maidstone. She was given a bottle of calcium SC. This involved placing a large needle under her skin and connecting to a so-called flutter valve which was a rubber tube with a hole at the top allowing air to bubble into the bottle above where it was plugged into the half-litre calcium bottle. It was always the student's job to hold the bottle high above your head, so gravity helped feed the fluid down. I heard the cow was up the next day.

Another week and it was time to get back to pathology, but the exams passed in both senses and I was back in the practice for the Easter "break".

I spent a lot of this seeing practice time with dogs and cat medicine and surgery. I assisted on many ops but had only just walked through the prep room on my way to the operating theatre when it blew up. There was a great bang, and the shop window front of the theatre was blown out with the crash of broken glass. Stuart was standing in the laboratory entrance off the theatre in the other direction with a black charred cigarette still in his fingers. He had been busy all morning spaying female cats and castrating male ones using ether. A great gaseous anaesthetic but with the tremendous disadvantage of being inflammable and explosive. Just as I was approaching, he had a cat ready on the operating table prepared for a spay. He being a smoker had snuck into the laboratory for a quick puff of a cigarette and the ether in the air had exploded. He certainly got more than a puff.

Nobody was hurt, given the amount of glass scattered around Mr Crowhurst's parking space, luckily empty at the time. I had just started to walk through so was lucky but the nurse in the theatre and Stuart were extremely fortunate; even the cat was unscathed apart from a brown singe which the owners did not notice as it was a tortoiseshell, and some extra fur was clipped off for the spay. The operation went ahead, and a new window was put in the next day and ether ceased to be the practice's gaseous anaesthetic of choice.

That time in the practice was also memorable for another reason. Arnold Crowhurst (AC) was known throughout the county as an equine expert veterinary surgeon. He had a massive Ford, I think it was a Granada, which only just fitted into the car parking space. One day his driver was away and he called me in, pointed at the car keys on the desk and told me I could drive him for the day. AC was more famous for his grunts than for anything he ever said. So, when I asked was he sure and was I insured, he just grunted. Not sure what that meant, I picked up the car keys and went to the yard hoping to reverse out before he came out, but he just followed me and climbed into the back seat. I did about a 52-point turn getting out of the yard and we set off on his first visit. Directions were difficult as like JC he did not say where we were going but simply different tone grunts for left and right and a disgruntled grunt if I went wrong.

The day was going as well as could be expected when, driving through Leeds village, famous for its castle, an oncoming car left me nowhere to go and I sharply pulled in left. Unfortunately, at that point in Leeds there is not a kerb but a great big embankment to the pavement. There was a horrid crunching noise and AC jumped out to check for damage. I was not sure whether to get out, but he soon jumped back in and said, "Great Danes," so knowing the hotel I turned left out of Leeds towards the hotel. "No, you've missed the turning." He meant go into Leeds Castle as he had to see Lady Bailey's Great Danes. This meant just entering the roundabout and leaving at the entrance road to double back on ourselves towards Leeds.

AC hated treating dogs, even ones as big as a horse, and just looked at the one presented to him by one of Lady Bailey's men and grunted "Get Jones"; neither the servant nor I knew what he was talking about but then I suddenly clicked he was suggesting his junior partner Richard Jones (RJ) should see the dog. We very quickly got back in the car and off to see some horses. He looked at several, mostly looking over the stable door and grunting at the owners who certainly seemed more subservient than Lady Bailey's servant. His instructions were to say the least succinct: "Put it out to grass", "Put a thicker rug on", "Feed more nuts" or "She is fine". Any questions of clarification were just met with a grunt.

In no time we were back at the practice and I had a chance to check the car for damage. It was unscathed and it was probably a tyre and hubcap that made the horrid noise on the wall, but I noticed Arnold drove himself home that night while I went to watch the evening surgery consultations. AC's driver was off all week so I had the privilege of driving him the rest of the week but learnt to look in the diary and at the map so I would not need too many directions.

The one time he did examine a horse was when he wanted to feel the tendons and prognosticate on recovery times from an injury. He would grunt, "Superficial tendon strain six weeks rest", "Deep tendon strain three months rest", and more sinister deep suspensory problems

"Turn out for a year or fire". By "fire" he was a believer in putting red hot needles into tendons to encourage scarring, a procedure now banned for the cruel procedure it was but even AC was honest enough to say he was not sure if firing worked, but it did enforce rest. Fifty years later AC has been proven correct: rest is the answer to tendon injuries in horses.

As AC suggested, RJ was a brilliant dog and cat clinician and we could not look at a case without him asking me to list the possible causes of vomiting in a dog or excess thirst in a cat. I clearly remember a springer spaniel peeing blood. He was so logical and thorough. Temperature, pulse, breathing rate, check lymph glands, listen to heart, check teeth and gums, feel abdomen, feel testes. Take detailed history from owner. Pass catheters, take urine sample, rectal examination. Make a diagnosis. He has a very enlarged prostate. We should x-ray him and run some bloods. If it is just benign prostatic enlargement you can castrate him or use female hormones to reduce the prostate. If more sinister and malignant you have a tough decision.

He prepared me very well for my final year at the Royal Veterinary College.

10

MEDICINE AND SURGERY

Both medicine and surgery were quite well taught at the RVC with a lot of hands-on experience. The small animal (SA – dog and cat) work was largely carried out in Camden Town at the charity Beaumont Hospital with clinics in which a small group of three or four of us would deal with both medical and surgical cases on a first opinion basis.

The farm work was mainly at the field station in Potters Bar but there was also some SA specialist medicine and surgery cases in which practitioners referred cases to the college specialists. There were some inherent difficulties with a shortage of common cattle, sheep or pig conditions for us students to deal with. Similarly, if common things occur commonly, these diseases were dealt with by the primary practices and the rare and obscure referred on to the college, giving us students a biased view of disease frequency.

For example, the commonest cause of lameness in cats is bite wound infection but the surgery department saw mainly rare orthopaedic problems of completely different cause. Very similarly, although we were taught that 80% of equine lameness was in the foot and usually caused by infection, I never saw a single equine lameness case at college due to infection. Poultry medicine was very well taught at the college farm and it needed to be as most general practices had no contact with the poultry industry.

My best decision in this last year was to live at the field station in Northumberland Hall of Residence. The fees were expensive per term, but it was well worth it: three-square meals a day, access to the library, access to the large animal (LA) hospital blocks and access to the SA hospital referral clinical cases. The only travelling we needed to do was one day a week to the Beaumont for first opinion cases, when we shared cars. This meant a lot more time to study as well as socialise.

One star character at both the Beaumont and at the field station was Mr Churchill-Frost, a bow-tie wearing surgeon whose main motto was to let nature take its course. Often when faced with a case, his line was, "What do we do? We do nothing, leave it alone. Don't touch it!" For example, a small cut on a dog's skin, which one of us had seen at the Beaumont: he would get the wound cleaned up and say his line, "What do we do? We do nothing, leave it alone. Don't touch it!" We very quickly learnt that some wounds were big enough to need suturing, but many were not. Those of us who had been to Professor Vaughan's orthopaedic lectures on anterior cruciate rupture in dogs would find one in the charity clinic and along would come C-F. He would agree with us on the diagnosis but say, "What do we do? We do nothing, leave it alone. Don't touch it!"

So, by finals we always knew there were two approaches: conservative or aggressive. Do nothing or wade in. For example, if the owners could afford the orthopaedic surgery on a big heavy young dog with a ruptured cruciate, then yes that was the best advice for the best outcome; but what if it were a charity case, a late middle-aged small lightweight dog, then, "What do we do? We do nothing, leave it alone. Don't touch it!" Or if the latter but overweight, the do nothing became get it to lose weight. Always in the non-surgical treatment of these sorts of cases, doing nothing did not mean neglecting cleaning wounds, antibiosis, and control of pain.

These dilemmas where no right or wrong are particularly important philosophical issues in veterinary medicine and we must always be reminded that because something can be done does not mean it necessarily should be done. These days we still talk of gold standard options where money no object, budget options and welfare reasons to consider euthanasia. These realities were emphasised at college, but it seems that vet college is still not the place where the harsh realities are in place and most graduates still want to offer only gold standard and feel if the client cannot afford it the practice should. C-Fs philosophy has, perhaps, been forgotten. Perhaps it is better understood if instead of gold standard we talk of Rolls-Royce. "How many clients can afford a Rolls Royce?" The rise of pet insurance has helped clients afford the unaffordable, but premiums can be eye-watering or the terms very constrictive.

The procedure with all medical investigations is: case history, signalment (species, age, breed and sex), signs and symptoms, clinical examination (temperature, pulse, stethoscope examination, etc.), differential diagnosis (all the possible causes of the problem), working diagnosis (the most likely cause of the problem), tests (to prove diagnosis using diagnostic aids such as ECG, blood tests, etc.), diagnosis (the actual cause of the disease). Finally, treatment (where possible), then outcome (what happens including if death a post-mortem – PM – and further PM tests).

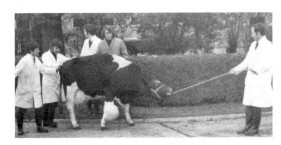

The above pattern is true of all medical cases – human, large animal or small. If in the above the treatment is surgery, the case becomes a surgical one.

A cattle case during final year at the RVC

I remember a bovine (cattle) cardiac case that my medicine group had to deal with, and I wrote up for my case book. It was what is called a case of "Traumatic Pericarditis".

Unlike rabbits and horses which are single stomached and rely on massive great large bowels to break down the cellulose of plants, cattle and sheep rely on multiple stomachs. That is why they are called ruminants. Cattle can sometimes swallow metal objects when grazing and these gravitate to the lowest stomach, the reticulum. If the metal object is sharp it can penetrate the stomach wall causing traumatic reticulitis, translated as injury-related inflammation of the stomach. If the penetration goes far enough forward, the lining sac surrounding the heart (pericardium) is affected, so-called pericarditis. Remember the suffix "-itis" means inflammation. So, the history of our case was a stunted underweight yearling purchased by the medical department. It was a castrated male Friesian yearling. It was underweight and in poor condition. On clinical examination it had a normal temperature, its pulse was weak, on stethoscope examination no heartbeat could be detected, its breathing rate was up, pinching at the top of its shoulders almost caused it to collapse, it was not chewing the cud normally and nothing abnormal was detected on rectal (back passage) examination. The differential diagnosis included all wasting diseases such as TB, cancers, etc., traumatic reticulitis and traumatic pericarditis.

The working diagnosis was traumatic pericarditis because of the withers pinch positive and lack of heart sounds, blood test results showed a high white cell count due to infection, ECG showed exceptionally low voltage waves due to fluid around the heart, needle drainage into cardiac area showed pus on drainage but a metal detector did not detect any wire in the stomach region. Finally, treatment: we considered further drainage of the pericardial area using larger needles and a stomach operation to remove the causative foreign body but previous attempts to treat these cases from research of clinical papers and texts and anecdotal stories from general practitioners had shown no success in this approach, so the poor beast was destroyed humanely, and post-mortem showed the heart sac full of pus, but no foreign body was found.

A sad but successfully diagnosed LA medical case following classic logical medical procedure.

11

EAST AFRICA

So, the summer approached, and it was time to head to East Africa in late June. The RAF had offered to fly the team out to Nairobi via Cyprus and we just had to all meet at RAF Brize Norton at 7am to fly out about 9am. I was staying in Berkeley, Gloucestershire, at the time as term had finished and invited a fellow team member, David, to stay the night. We were so excited about the trip that we chatted into the night and went to bed with no one for some reason setting an alarm.

We woke at 8.30 in a state of absolute panic, got dressed and rushed to a phone box at the end of the drive. We spoke to the control tower talking to the pilot of our Hercules with the rest of the team and equipment on board as he taxied down the runway. I thought that was the end of the trip for us unless we got a flight to Nairobi at our expense. The controller, however, just calmly told us they had other flights to Cyprus that day and come to Brize Norton as soon as possible. We grabbed a lift for the hour's drive to the air base and later that afternoon took off for Cyprus in a Belfast transport plane.

It was a massive plane with a big cargo to go to RAF Akrotiri. The flight was great, and the flight engineers were so kind to us apart from one who sat next to me in a row of seats for a while, buckled himself in and started chatting. Somehow, I suppose inevitably, the conversation got to the recent Trident plane crash near Heathrow earlier that month (18th June 1972) killing all 118 on board. He explained it crashed due to a stall, and once it had stalled took 30 seconds to hit the ground. "Thirty seconds is a long time when you know you are going to die," he mused, looking at his watch. He counted out 30 seconds "30…29…28…"; by the time he got to zero I had stopped breathing. He tapped me on the knee and said, "Good job Belfasts are very safe," as he undid his seat belt, jumped up and attended to his duties, leaving me a shivering wreck gasping for breath.

It has taken me several long-haul flights to Australia when sitting in a jet for almost a day to cure me of the fear of flying that member of the RAF installed in me, having flown fearlessly during RAF camps with the ATC. When we landed and were reunited with Bob and the team, I expected a telling off, but he was in fact exceedingly kind saying he would have funded flights as we were both important members of the team, and then he praised us for blagging the flight the way we had because the RAF had been very non-committal about even the original Hercules flight until the last moment.

I then accompanied him to the manifest desk to check on our flight to Nairobi the next day.

While Bob was busy, I recognised a fellow member from the ATC and school at one of the manifest desks. I shouted, "Hey Pollard." He looked down his nose when greeted by a long-haired student. "Flying Officer Pollard to you," he said, before recognising me. David Pollard had obviously signed up after school and fulfilled his dream of going to RAF Cranwell. He was immediately less pompous than his greeting and picked me up in his car an hour later when he had finished. He was very enthusiastic saying, "I think I've got you a flight in a fighter jet," as I jumped in his sports car, an MG, and tore off. I was slightly less enthusiastic after my conversation with the flight engineer. As luck would have it, he could not arrange it at the last minute and he thought my sigh of relief was a sigh of disappointment. The tour of the base was remarkably interesting; then we met up with the rest of the team in the officers' mess for a drink. They were not only impressed that David and I had made it to Cyprus, they were also impressed with my contact from school, Flying Officer Pollard.

The next day Flying Officer Pollard saw us off on another Hercules, a different one and this time with the whole team on board.

It was dark when we landed in Nairobi and I remember driving through the shanty towns we had seen as we landed. We were greeted by Bob's Nairobi contact, Jack, a great character who took us under his wing and found accommodation for the whole team. He had even bought a minibus for the team as Bob had requested. I think most of the team were put up at the university, but Ellis and me and a couple of others were lodged with our host. Anyway, I spent that evening having a great lasagne at the Nairobi Hilton and a visit to a night club he had shares in. We spent a fantastic week in Nairobi while Bob and most of the team sorted out the logistics of the brucella testing that needed to be done at the university once we got back from Uganda.

The week in Nairobi was well spent from my point of view, touring our host's businesses in the city and enjoying the live band at his night club whilst the newly purchased minibus was serviced at one of our host's contacts.

Robin and I were asked to drive the minibus to Nakuru and collect some of our equipment which had been stored there. We were going to meet some friends of Jack's at Nakuru and stay the night on their farm, where some of the team were already staying. I hoped to see some of Kenya's wildlife on the drive, but nothing was sighted. Bob and the rest of the team were staying as guests of Bob's girlfriend Anthea at her parent's farm at the neighbouring town of Naivasha, which was our first stop.

After a busy few days with little time to explore the beautiful area, Robin and I were asked to drive the bus from Nairobi to Entebbe in Uganda. We were incredibly happy to be asked to do this but were told to be wary of the Ugandan army guards at the border. It was a 10-hour drive and we planned to set off early and try and get the 535km (about 330 miles) drive done in a day. The rest of the team were going to fly to Entebbe from Nairobi. I had not realised Bob had regarded flying most of the team in rather than at least a minibus full of us going by road as safer because of the likelihood of border problems if we turned up mob-handed. I was also surprised that we were only asked to take a little equipment and the Weetabix that had been donated by the company when I wrote to them on my worn-out typewriter.

Ignorance is bliss, they say, but I was hearing more and more from our new Kenyan friends of the Ugandan dictator, Idi Amin, and his out-of-control army. I was surprised by two things on the drive: firstly, pleasantly by the quality of the roads, and secondly and sadly, that I had been in Africa over a week and still not seen any game. I offered to share the driving, but Robin told me Bob had been adamant that only he could drive. I wondered what my purpose was. "You're shotgun," Robin said – and laughed. When we arrived at the border town of Busia we were greeted by Kenyan border patrol; without question they lifted the barrier and we drove two hundred yards to a sign that said "Busia Border Uganda".

Very stern-faced armed and uniformed men told us to get out of the vehicle and sent us into a nearby boiling-hot hut. Behind a desk sat a soldier in uniform and by the door was another – both were armed with rifles. The man sat behind the desk looked at Robin and me as if we were certainly up to no good. Bob had given us some money and told us to fill up with petrol before the border. He took all our personal money. He said to hide the rest in the bus but put two of the biggest notes in each of our passports for the border. The army officer put his feet up on the desk alongside his rifle next to an unguarded electric fan blowing at him alone and said one word, "Passport". He looked at them a long time: I did not notice where the money went. He threw the passports back at me. "All you whites look alike to me," he said. I made the mistake of laughing as Robin was tall with blond hair and I was shorter and dark-haired. He removed his feet from the desk and in an instant the rifle was pointing at us.

It was then I heard the loudest click I have heard in my life as he switched the safety catch off. I noticed the armed soldier at the door move round out of the line of fire. He asked why we were coming to Uganda. I said it was for research for his government on cow diseases, and in unbelievably bad Swahili: "Daktari ya gombe," – cow doctor. "Have you any more money?" "No," I replied, remembering my weapons training that a gun is always loaded, never point it unless at a target and always assume the safety catch is off. I was sure this man could not read from his perusing the passports, but I was sure the safety catch was off. The world stood still and the electric fan on his desk stopped, or appeared to, and he gave a sort of smile through broken teeth. He switched the rifle safety catch back on with a quieter click and I picked up the passports and we backed out of the office. The barrier was lifted, and we were in Uganda.

We stopped up the road shaking, and Robin said, "I bet that rifle was not loaded."

"The gun is always loaded," I told him, looking under the rear carpet where I had put the rest of the money, "and the money has gone." The Weetabix supply for the team had also gone.

The roads varied between tarmac and dirt, but we made good time to the Victoria Hotel in Entebbe to meet Bob who was exceedingly pleased to see us and the minibus. I told him of our brush with the army and the loss of his money and the Weetabix. "Of course they took it when they searched the bus." I asked why Bob, if not insured to drive, picked me to accompany Robin?

"I knew the border would be tricky and you have such an innocent face." He laughed when I told him that to Ugandan soldiers we all look the same. The whole team stayed a short time at a government hostel near the airport down the road from the Victoria Entebbe Airport Hotel. We collected four Dodge trucks supplied by foreign aid, arranged by Bob, and the team split in two, half going in two Dodges to Mbarara and the other two Dodges and the minibus going to the Karamoja region. In Mbarara we would be doing cattle parasitic worm counts and cultures and brucellosis testing and in Karamoja TB and brucellosis testing.

I was assigned to Mbarara. We stayed in what can only be described as Hopper Huts on a ranch outside of the main town with a cookhouse dining area under a long, corrugated-iron roof with ten rooms with two camp beds in each. The toilet facilities were a shed built around a pit with a bank of toilet seats. We called it the "long drop". The highlight of our facility was the fully-equipped mobile caravan laboratory which had been parked there just before we arrived. We soon settled to a daily routine of driving to a farm ranch or government communal tick dip once or twice a day and collecting blood and dung samples. The blood samples were stored for later brucella testing and the dung samples had worm egg counts done and we incubated them, identifying some of the worm species from their eggs and the rest from their larvae.

As I say, our ranch was out of town and all trips to town involved driving past the Mbarara barracks which was always done with trepidation as the guards looked at our trucks suspiciously. The local cattle breeds we worked on were long-horned Ankole which had a sort of buffalo features, Brahmans, the Indian breed, and some more recognisable Hereford or Friesian crosses. Overall, the local tribesmen brought roughly five or six cattle at a time to the local dips; they were tame and managed easily in stocks. The government ranches' cattle were wilder, especially the Brahmans, but the ranches usually had good cattle handling facilities, generally modern crushes.

On the way back from one of the government farms we came across an army roadblock formed by a truck parked across the road and six soldiers all pointing rifles at us. Those of us sat in the back of the truck stood as one of the soldiers approached our lead Dodge. As the driver, Guy, opened his door the soldier saw the Ugandan coat of arms with the crested crane emblazoned on the driver's door panel showing they were government trucks. The soldier quickly accepted our explanation that we were working for the government on animal health and the soldiers moved off the road and waved us through.

Later that same week, since the project was going so well and the roadblock had waved us through, we felt brave enough to head into town, which meant driving past the barracks after dark. We all joined the local tennis, golf and social club and for once I was pleased not to be a designated driver on the trucks and, as I said, the minibus had gone to the northern project. The locals in the club were very friendly, including Europeans, Asians and Africans, and the memberships were initially equally divided between the three groups. The beer and banter flowed, and we all had a great time after being accepted as temporary members.

One night at the club the beer flowed more than usual, and I was invited to stay for a couple after our sober driver got a bit bored and ready to go home. I was invited to stay and be put up by a couple who taught science in the local school. They offered me a lift back to our camp the following day, a Saturday, if I promised to show them around our mobile lab. I easily agreed to this and had a couple more Tusker beers until spending the night at their lovely house next to the club.

In the middle of the night, I awoke with my bladder full from the beers and opened the French doors out to their garden and went into the beautiful moonlit garden; coming in through a different door I wandered down a long corridor and found the toilet at the end. By this time, I was bursting so imagine my surprise when on emerging from the toilet I saw puddles all the way down the corridor and the puddles smelt of urine. Fearing I had embarrassed myself, I spent ten minutes mopping the corridor with loo paper when a very friendly but large German Shepherd dog wandered past me as I knelt wiping up and cocked his leg three more times down the now clean corridor. The next morning, I did not have either the heart nor the head to discuss my nocturnal problems or their much-loved dog's lack of house training.

During our time there, each weekend four of our team were given the weekend to go travelling. My four included the team's scientific leader, Pete, and Brenda and Fred. We decided to hire a car in town and drive to Queen Elizabeth game park as none of us had seen any African wildlife during our month's stay in East Africa. The park was two hours' drive from Mbarara but mostly on unmade roads, except we missed the entrance to the park and went about an hour out of our way. We picked up a local African in a big red shirt walking down the road and gave him a lift. He promised to direct us and sat in the back with Brenda and Fred. We dropped him at his village and he pointed the way to the park – looking at the map we suspected we had gone even further out of our way to drop him off. I was driving and Pete was in the passenger seat with Brenda and Fred in the back; it was only later that an embarrassed Brenda told us the shirt was the only thing that our friend was wearing! Fred had not noticed.

We arrived at the park at dusk and rather than stay in the campsite decided to splash out for our first night in the lodge but not until after we had driven around a magnificent herd of buffalo. I was told they can be the most aggressive but the herd we went through seemed calm. The next morning, we discovered the starter motor on our hire car was a bit hit and miss but was easily bump started and we were on our safari tour of the park. We saw the famous tree climbing lions with one posing in a tree for us. Warthogs, baboons and herds of elephants were spotted on our first drive. We were a little nervous when we stopped, remembering not to turn off the engine as nobody fancied push-starting in a pride of Lions.

Towards the end of the morning drive, we were back near the lodge looking at the large herd of buffalo when I stalled the car. After several turns of the ignition, we just got the ominous whirring click of the starter. We all sat frozen. "I'm not getting out," Fred said.

But after five minutes the bull was becoming more curious and some of the cows were close to the car. Now or never, I said, and jumped out of the car with just the flimsy door as my shield and pushed, holding on to the steering wheel. The others took my prompt and jumped out and pushed, Pete and Brenda even brave enough to push from the boot. As the car gained momentum, I jumped in, depressed the clutch, had the ignition on and engaged second gear. She started first time, leaving the two brave boot pushers stranded in the herd. They quickly jumped in and we were off. In the afternoon we drove to the creek and saw hippopotamuses and in the main river at a good distance with the engine running, Nile crocodiles.

That afternoon we pitched our tent in the campsite and as we did an elephant wandered to the camp bin area and started to rattle around the bins. Our respect for the wildlife was foremost in our minds but not so for one camper who saw it as a perfect photo opportunity, getting far too close to the scavenging loner who was a young bull. He suddenly charged the photographer and covered half the distance between them in an instant. The photographer dropped his awfully expensive camera and ran as fast as he could but the distance to the elephant shrank; fortunately, a few yards from his target the elephant stopped and stamped the ground, ears flapping. He then turned back to his bins and only after he left did the photographer retrieve his dusty, dirty, and probably damaged camera.

What a day we'd had and we decided to eat at the lodge just a few hundred yards from the campsite. Our adventures were not over because as we walked back the buffalo were grazing between us and the campsite, so we skirted around them. The African sky on a clear night is awesome and we spent some time sitting outside our tent looking up, listening to the noisy insects. Pete and Brenda had a one-person tent each but I was sharing with Fred: the roaring lions sounded like they were just outside the tent. The next morning Fred woke me and said he was extremely hot. I reminded him he had on the thickest winceyette pyjamas both top and bottom. He took the top off and soon woke me again saying how hot he still was. Perspiration was pouring off him. I quickly got dressed and asked him if he had taken his anti-malarial tablet. Yes, he said, every day and I believed him.

We soon drove and tracked down a local African doctor who agreed Fred had malaria and gave him an antimalarial injection using an old silver syringe and needle set. Thank goodness this was pre-HIV. Fred rallied and by the afternoon we had one more magnificent game drive, again seeing the tree lions, including one male with a black mane that the park was famous for. We had at last seen Africa. Fred eventually needed treatment for repeat bouts of malaria over the next few years at the Hospital for Tropical Diseases in London.

We went back to work with renewed vigour and got into a great routine blood testing the cattle and collecting hundreds of dung samples which I incubated for worm larvae after egg counting. If we got behind with the lab work, I would let the others go sampling while I stayed and caught up with it.

One day when I did go sampling, we were at a tick dip and met up with a local African vet. He told us a great story about the tick dip we were at. He said the cattle around there started dying of tick fever and the tick infestation in the cattle did not seem very controlled. He told the young new dip station supervising officer to throw another can of dip into the tank where the cattle jumped in to dip them. The next month the problem was worse so he repeated his instructions: "Throw in another can of dip." When the problem got worse, the Veterinary Officer ordered the tank drained and at the bottom of the dip were 12 canisters of dip – all unopened. The young dip station officer had only ever been told to throw the cans in; nobody had ever told him that really meant taking the lids off and pouring the liquid in the tank. The poor lad assumed the cans dissolved and he had done exactly as he had been told but at what cost to the tick control scheme.

I also paid the price for visiting a tick area and was shocked the next morning in the shower to see a little gold tick on my manhood. I rushed into the kitchen for matches, then went into the long drop, striking a match hoping there was not too much methane about and blew it out, then with surgical precision and no shaky hand touched it on the parasite that immediately let go and dropped off. I had spent my whole time in Africa in shorts and it must have crawled up from the long grass near the tick dip as we were sampling the cattle.

Ticks find their host by crawling up plants and hanging off leaves with their legs reaching forward, a process known as questing. They then have a blood meal from the host to lie dormant on the ground or lay eggs which hatch larval forms until the next questing stage of their life cycle. I had inadvertently become a host in the most unlikely eye-watering of anatomical places. The drop into the pit meant one tick at least would not complete its life cycle.

During our time in Mbarara we managed two more safaris: one to Murchison Falls and another to see the gorillas. Murchison falls was a six-hour drive from Mbarara but worth every bone-shaking moment.

It is where the Nile flows through a gorge just over 20ft wide (6m) and then plunges over 140 feet, producing a spectacular waterfall. I have never seen Victoria Falls or Niagara Falls but Murchison with its little footpath down alongside the falls would certainly take my vote with its noise and spectacular scenery and energy. Just down river from Murchison is the country's largest population of Nile crocodiles which are amazing and the boat trip we did to see them also allowed viewings of many elephant families and solitary ones at the waterside and deep in the water showering. There was also a substantial hippopotamus population.

Our trip to see the gorillas was Paul's idea. I had done my farm project with him and we were based together in the Mbarara team. Spontaneously, one weekend he suggested we all get into one truck and head to the Rwandan border area where the mountain gorillas live. We headed to Bwindi, a two-hundred-mile round trip, but when we got to the lodge nobody was around. We finally found a little old lady who opened the lodge and served us all tea, but she said no guides were available and they were all on an anti-poaching trip. It was a spectacular drive but, in the end, fruitless as we did not see the gorillas in our midst.

It was now late August 1972 and the political situation in the country was deteriorating; perhaps that is the real reason the menfolk were not around. In early August President Amin had said that Britain would need to take responsibility for the British Asians, accusing them of sabotaging the country's economy and corruption. It was obvious to us that it was the Asians who in fact drove the economy forwards, but Amin was finding the classic internal scapegoat for all the country's ills. Alongside the anti-British Asian sentiment there was a growing generalised anti-British sentiment. Within a week the policy of British Asian expulsion was expanded to include all citizens of India, Pakistan and Bangladesh.

During our trips to farms there were more roadblocks and more aggressive interrogations of our team members by the army including, "Where had we stolen the trucks from?"

At this stage I was at the camp more and more to try to get our cultures and egg counts sorted before, as British passport holders, we were to be expelled. Things deteriorated rapidly and one night there was much more noise coming from the Mbarara barracks as we drove by and no armed guards outside. When we arrived at the club there were no Asian or African members to be seen, just a surly African sitting at the bar without a drink. I did not recognise him as a member. The Europeans who were there warned us he was from the government and obviously keeping an eye on us. I tried my usual friendly approach and offered him a drink, but he declined. Stupidly I bought a whisky and put it in front of him. He looked very stern but did not make eye contact. A short time later I saw him surreptitiously drinking the whisky straight and that his hand was shaking. I realised he was more scared than us. We made a quick exit and as we went by the barracks it was even noisier again with no guards and it seemed every soldier in the barracks was drunk.

The next day Bob made the sensible decision to pull the plug on the research projects and get out of Uganda. We all headed to the accommodation near Entebbe airport and handed back the trucks and luckily there were no roadblocks between Mbarara and Entebbe. Within a day or so we were all in Entebbe. The team members in the Karamoja had also got some good work done but it seemed food was harder to come by as they had all lost weight. Bob set about getting us all flights back to Nairobi and arranging air transportation for our brucella blood samples so they could be tested in Nairobi University.

It meant a few days of freedom and I went one night to the Entebbe Airport Hotel where I was invited to join a BA crew in transit overnight for a meal and several drinks. I was sitting next to the captain but I was, of course, more interested in the gorgeous hostesses. As the evening wore on, he offered me a drink in his room, but I declined and continued chatting and drinking with the hostesses. I did not even consider it a proposition. This was, of course, the 1970s. I stayed up with the crew until about 2am when I thought I had better head back to our accommodation. I walked out of the hotel and was walking around the airport road with the perimeter fence to my right.

I was about half-way home when I heard a truck behind me. I dived into the bush and lay flat on my belly. It was as I feared a military patrol. They had stepped these up with the recent troubles, and I am not sure if my hiding was a good idea. As they drove by it was obvious I was not the only one who had had a drink that night: the armed soldiers in the back of the truck were shouting and waving their rifles and arms in the air. I saw how dangerous the alternative option of continuing to walk down the road could have led to a very life-threatening incident given the current attitude to the British. On the other hand, I realised if I had been spotted lying in the bush I would have been accused of spying because the Ugandan Air Force jets were kept at Entebbe Airport.

When I first heard the excited shouts as they drove by, I thought someone had seen me, but they were so close I could see the one holding a bottle was glassy-eyed in the lorry light hanging in the back of the truck and I waited until they were long gone before climbing out of the bush and hurrying home. I had entered Uganda a carefree boy and was leaving it a politically aware man. Knowing if one mad man shot Amin, we would all be massacred, whereas back home in England the Houses of Parliament could be blown up and the Royal family killed but somehow the British Constitution would survive with the next in line to the throne taking over and a new government formed.

Not so in most parts of the world, particularly Uganda in 1972. I spent the next few days by the pool at the hotel but always made sure I was back in our accommodation before dark.

We flew back to Nairobi by a flight from Entebbe, except Pete who got an earlier than planned Aeroflot flight home via Moscow.

When we arrived in Nairobi it seemed that Kenya had got as jumpy and nervously anti-British as the Ugandans. About half the group were not given visas to stay the two weeks in Kenya: we were meant to wait for our RAF flights home but had to get flights straight home. I was lucky and was granted a visa and a group of us headed back to Nakuru after sorting out the work that needed to be done at the University of Nairobi on the blood samples. David stayed there and organised this. My laboratory work on my part of the project was finished before leaving Uganda. As a result, it was just a question of waiting to see if and when we got our RAF flight.

The crisis in Uganda and East Africa meant more RAF flights but whether there would be room for us on a flight home as scheduled was, no pun intended, "up in the air". I had a fantastic time visiting Lake Naivasha with its variety of game including zebra and Lake Nakuru with its sea of pink flamingos while staying as a guest of Jack's friend Susan. We were taken on a trip to the Rift Valley museum, showing the Leakey family's work on the evolution of man with Australopithecus species and early Homo species all found nearby. That afternoon we drove to a tea plantation at Kericho and saw the tea hedges growing.

We had just sat down to afternoon tea when a chair on the neighbouring table was thrown back and the gentleman sitting in it crashed to the floor and he lay prone. His wife and daughter screamed and ran off shouting he was dead. I felt for his pulse and could not feel one, he was ashen and not breathing. I turned him on his back and was about to start mouth-to-mouth and cardiac massage but first hit him firmly on his sternum. He sat up with a jolt and his colour returned and so more importantly did his pulse. His family gathered around and he was taken indoors. A local doctor soon examined him and confirmed that he had had another mild heart attack after landing in Nairobi the day before. Travelling to the altitude of the tea plantation had been too much for his frail circulation, but his family were grateful I was on the spot and felt a little ashamed of the way they had run away from a family member needing help.

The weekend before we were due to fly home, several of us were invited to play football in a team of Europeans against a local team. Four of us were picked up by the captain of the team in his Range Rover, the first time I had ridden in such a comfortable four-wheel drive vehicle, more used to the back of a Dodge truck. We drove to a little village a mile out of Nairobi and as there were twelve of us and just a few spectators, I volunteered to drop out and referee. The African team emerged from the changing room hut which looked genuinely like a bar and I was about to blow the whistle for the game to start when one by one about seven trucks arrived from surrounding villages, each full of about thirty supporters. They were very vocal and had obviously come from far and wide to see the match.

The game kicked off in more ways than one. The captain who had given me a lift was upended by one of the local team in a most violent way. I had a word with the tackler and got a smile back, but the truckloads of supporters heckled me. Within minutes the same player brought down another of the European side, much to the pleasure of the crowd. No yellow cards in those days but I did talk to him and went to take his number but there was not one. No more than five minutes later the same player kicked out at an opponent, grounding him with a blow to the shin. The crowd was chanting now, and I felt I had no choice but to send the offender off. I thought there was going to be a riot as the offender retired to the bar, but he was cheered off and then I realised I too was being cheered for being brave or stupid enough to send him off.

The eleven-man European side scored but then tired and the local side scored an equaliser, and the game ended a draw. Afterwards one of the local team came up to me and asked me to join his team in the bar. None of the Europeans were invited in: they were taken drinks out on the touchline. I walked into the dark bar which was tiny and there was the player I had sent off surrounded by his teammates. He shook hands, handed me a cold beer and apologised for his behaviour, saying he was carried away by the moment.

On the drive home we saw Jomo Kenyatta's personal motorcycle outriders just behind us; they were not in a motorcade, just heading somewhere for an official duty when a local drove his car into the convoy from a side road and knocked one of them off his motorbike. We pulled over and were horrified to witness all the bikes park, pull the careless driver out of his vehicle, and lay into him with their truncheons. I would like to think when they saw us pulled in a little ahead of them in a Range Rover, they would not kill the poor man, but they were still laying into him as we drove off feeling useless. Africa was still its cruel self.

It looked like the direct flight back from Nairobi to Brize Norton was going ahead and a few of us had one last night in Jack's night club. The flight did go ahead as planned with all our research results in the bag, given the political setbacks.

12

FINALS

In September 1972 it was back to college for the last two terms in which I had to finish my medicine and surgery case books, write the first draft of the Ugandan Parasitic Worm Project, then pass the written practical and oral final exams in both subjects as well as completing the 26 weeks of seeing practice in the Christmas break between the two terms.

I had to hit the ground running and made the obvious decision to stay at the Northumberland Hall of Residence based at the college field station. This allowed plenty of time after the academic day to get all the workload under control. I waded through all my notes, read all the latest American textbooks on both subjects and my UK textbooks were extremely well thumbed. I met up regularly with Pete to read through and re-draft my report on the Ugandan Cattle Project. It also gave me an insight into Pete's research work. He had got a PhD in sheep x goat hybrids and was still researching at his own unit at the Field Station, unlike crosses between horses and donkeys which produce the hybrid mule. The sheep-goat hybrid was non vital, leading to early embryo death, and Pete's scientific brain and knowledge were second to none.

The research teams work together resulted in the publication in the *British Veterinary Journal* of our paper entitled "Helminthiasis in the Ankole District of Uganda". Pete and Bob's modesty insisted I was the lead author, and the rest of the team was listed as "et al". I also got co-authorship of the two other scientific publications resulting from our Ugandan work on "TB and Brucellosis in Cattle in the Karamoja region of Uganda". Two papers written by David and Pete but again

Pete and Bob insisted David got lead authorship.

Once the final drafts were submitted to the respective journals it was a waiting game for final publication. All in all, the work we did in Uganda was extremely useful, but I suspect any veterinary advance helping the animal and human population was negated by Idi Amin's extremes and a further civil war in the next few years.

During the winter term of final year there was a Men's 15 v. Ladies Rugby Match in which the RVC first fifteen played against all the college ladies – and what was a fun event nearly turned into a tragedy. I went home that weekend so missed the match but Ian who I went to Yugoslavia with did play. He was a regular for both the college and London University and was the best player in the college. Nobody thought anything of the fact he scored a try near the posts despite at least 20 ladies trying to stop him and eight of them trapping him against the goalpost as he touched the ball down.

It was only afterwards when he passed out in the showers and felt unwell that some of his teammates were worried. Ian went back to his flat for an early night. Thank goodness one of his flatmates, Mike, was a final-year medical student and found him unconscious in the corridor in the early hours of the morning and diagnosed internal bleeding. He was rushed to hospital and given a blood transfusion and an emergency splenectomy. The best player in the college and perhaps the University of London at the time had ruptured his spleen playing rugby against ladies.

He had been admitted to Highgate Hospital for his treatment and towards the end of his stay half a dozen of us in white coats, stethoscopes in hand, paid him a visit. Hospital security was very lax. We arrived at his bedside and pulled the curtains around the bed. Ian was feeling much better but was in danger of bursting his stitches from laughing too much – as a team he knew to be vet students were getting away with impersonating doctors. One of the nurses came to investigate and she saw the funny side of things and saw that, although a little yellow, so did Ian.

The next thing he was bundled into a wheelchair and taken on a tour of the hospital. We got in the lift and did a visit to every ward and the white coats and stethoscopes gave us access to all areas, much to the amusement of most of the patients when we whispered that we were vets checking up on a colleague. Amazingly there were no repercussions and Ian was discharged to our, or rather his, flatmates' care in a couple of days.

As well as the studying, I also contributed one joke sketch to the final-year review. I was reminded how I spent almost as much time in the pathology museum and specimen room before the last exams as I had in front of the Eclipse skeleton in the anatomy room. Almost half those pathological specimens were tuberculosis lesions of various organs. So, my sketch was a "viva voce", the so-called practical oral exam literally translated as spoken exam simply known as vivas. In the sketch the student is handed a preserved specimen by one of the lecturers and the student says, "TB or not TB, that is the question?"

The whole show went well, and it was the end of term in a few days. It was straight back to my foster practice for me. So much had changed since my last stay. JC had left the partnership to set up his own practice in Leicestershire. RJ had virtually given up dog and cat work and was concentrating on horses as AC was doing a little less. A new dog and cat partner, Janet, was joining the partnership and Stuart was still there. The practice was as busy as ever and I was allowed to do so many procedures. I became expert at dog, cat, cattle, sheep and horse intravenous injections (IV) as well as the easier intramuscular (IM) and under skin (SC).

I was even allowed to do surgery completing, while supervised, a dog and a cat female neutering or "spay" as it was known, and the male neutering equivalent obviously called castrations. I had previously castrated male piglets with JC, now I completed the set with dog, cat, cattle, sheep and horse castrations. Many pet owners, especially male owners, are uncomfortable with the thought of neutering their pets, especially not surprisingly male ones. The benefits of castration with male cats are obvious: toms spend so much of their time wandering a wide territory fighting other male cats that bite wounds are common.

They are also difficult to house train and tend to spray their pungent urine around any territory, including the home. Eventually as they mature, they get that tom cat smell which is as smelly as the urine. The benefits of neutering male dogs are more debatable, but it obviously makes them infertile, less likely to sexual wandering looking for a mate or pursuing the scent of an in-season bitch. It can help produce beneficial behaviour changes. They are also less likely to have prostatic problems in later life, less likely to have hormone-driven tumours of the bottom and obviously no chance of testicular cancer as they have been removed.

The main benefit of spaying female dogs (bitches) and cats (queens) is that they cannot breed but it also stops them coming into season and for cats that means noisy calling for the tom and very strange rolling behaviour. This is because in the usual form of the operation the ovaries and womb are surgically removed.

I was also allowed to carry out many vaccinations of puppies, kittens and adult dogs and cats. The disease prevented in cats was one caused by a parvovirus called panleucopaenia, a virus that attacks any rapidly growing cells and was a real killer of unvaccinated kittens and young cats. We would see at least a case a week; they would be presented by their owners weak and dehydrated and the mortality rate was 90% plus with an occasional, usually older cat pulling through but only after intensive nursing and fluid therapy. The dogs were vaccinated for two types of leptospirosis (Weil's disease and dog lepto) – remember the coypu. The dogs were also vaccinated for distemper, a virus related to measles virus in children that attacks the gut of dogs but also the nervous system, so we saw the acutely vomiting cases with diarrhoea and a week or so later if they survived signs of nervous problems, wobbly movement, inco-ordination, or fitting.

During that winter I also saw cases about once a week including the "hardpad" form of the disease where the chronic recovered dogs had thickened pads and they could be heard stomping down the corridor with their thick soles and nervous problems. Many that made it through this far still had to be put to sleep. Euthanasia was one of the commonest reasons for dog or cat consultations and owners of both dogs and cats on this sad occasion were strangely proud that their 13-year-old dog or their 10-year-old cat "had never seen a vet its whole life".

Widespread vaccination to prevent the common diseases and a more caring attitude means these days it is much rarer to hear such comments.

As I say, euthanasia was a common consultation appointment and as my IV technique improved I could carry out the procedure. It involved the injection of 5-40ml of concentrated barbiturate but always only after a long assessment of quality of life and discussion with the owner by the vet I was with, be it Stuart or Janet. This is the saddest job carried out by a vet and even after all my time in practice it generates personal hurt and sadness wrapped in an envelope of professional pride if it goes well, which it usually does.

I also honed my farm and equine skills during this Christmas period and quickly realised how I loved this outside work in the summer but was a different story in the middle of winter. Stuart did a calving of a beautiful Hereford cow in a dark cold shed but even with both of us in a parturition gown it was freezing. Stuart had placed a head rope and invited me to place the two-foot ropes above the fetlocks or wrist joints. The calf was obviously alive as it moved when I felt the rope around the back of its head behind its ears and round and in its mouth. The foot ropes were soon in place and my hand and arm was warming inside the cow.

With the three ropes in place, Stuart showed me how to wrap them around a sawn third of a pickaxe handle without knotting, no matter how hard the handle was pulled. The farmer pulled one leg and I pulled the other with Stuart pulling the head. As the cow was standing, he reminded us to pull downwards as the calf literally dived out of the cow but needed help with the strength of three of us. The cow's head was held by the farmer's daughter and we worked as a team. Stuart did another internal, easing the calf's head with his hand as I pulled on the head rope this time. Then we all returned to our respective ropes and pulled hard as the front legs appeared one in front of the other, then the head and in a rush the whole calf.

Stuart and I lifted the calf's hind end over a gate, and he massaged his chest as he started breathing; I say he because I was told by the farmer's daughter it was a bull calf. On Stuart's instructions I did another internal examination on the cow, warm hands again, to check for internal injuries and that there was not a second calf. I took this opportunity to also put some antibiotic pessaries in her. The afterbirth had come out straight after the calf which was good news. This would be another good case for my surgical case book.

Staying at the practice that night had been worth it. Stuart had cooked a great meal before we got called out and I sadly remember his girlfriend loudly vomiting in the toilet as we left on the call. Nobody had a drink as we were on duty so I was surprised. He said she had an eating disorder. That was the first time I had heard or witnessed Bulimia nervosa and it was such a shock. It took the edge of a successful evening.

A few nights later I was invited to stay at RJ's as he was on duty. We had a lovely home-cooked meal by his wife Sue and were chatting when the phone rang. It was the police. There was a horse on the A20 nearby that had been hit by a car. We jumped in the car and less than a couple of miles away we saw the police car and a badly smashed mini.

The windscreen was shattered and the roof severely dented. The driver was shocked but unhurt and talking to the police. We were told the horse was up the bank by the side of the road lying in some undergrowth. As we approached, she "stood up". I grabbed her head collar, and we were both shocked to see she was not in fact standing but had fractured both her forelimbs above the fetlock, just where I had placed the calving ropes on the Hereford bull calf. The lovely bay thoroughbred mare had simply dug her compound fracture stumps into the soft earth. The policeman arrived with a strong torch that illuminated the full horror as she fell back down with her stumps pointing down the slope. RJ had not got a gun, but two bottles of the dog barbiturates intravenously quickly put her out of her misery, and we went back to RJ's saddened, but he was professional enough to ring the knacker or hunt who were going to collect the mare and reminded them they could not do anything other than move the mare next day, as an owner needed to be found and, as barbiturates had been used, the horsemeat could not be fed to hounds. The driver of the car was in fact so lucky to have survived a head-on collision with the horse whilst behind the steering wheel of a mini. It was so close to a double tragedy.

I had Christmas Day and Boxing Day off then back to the practice before New Year again, staying with RJ at his home and Stuart in the flat over the surgery. I calculated I would just clock my 26 weeks seeing practice by the time I was due back at the RVC. So apart from passing medicine and surgery written papers, practical and viva, I would be in practice by, appropriately, April Fool's Day.

The next and last term began and even in late January everyone was already a little tense. As far as practical ability was concerned, so much depended on the quality of the foster practice and how much they let their students do. Personally, I had no worries about the hands-on techniques and more worried about the academic details. Had I read enough theory? Did I know all the latest papers in the vet journals? Nonetheless, I kept up with both the large and small animal medical and surgical referrals that came in day and night but to be honest there were just a couple of broken nights with equine colic surgeries and one calving which was really an abortion investigation as the young heifer gave birth to a premature, bald, deformed, rotting calf and needed a little help.

The dog and cat referrals were mainly during normal hours and I remember a dog with a slipped disc heading for surgery and we were told to do a pre-op examination. I told the lecturer that I thought the dog had a low-grade heart murmur and only after a careful stethoscope examination he reluctantly agreed. This stimulated my embryonic interest in cardiology, especially when the medical houseman was called, and he agreed with me, although successful spinal surgery went ahead after early mitral valve disease (MVD) was confirmed. Not sure if I got a feather in my cap from the medical department or a black mark from the surgical department for the delay I had caused.

The examinations loomed and one of my main interests, preventive medicine, had a paper to itself. The logic seemed obvious to me: to prevent disease, what can be done? Firstly, improve genetics, some strains and breeds are more resistant to illness and disease than others. Secondly, nutrition, a balanced diet was important with enough of each food building block – protein, fat, carbohydrates, minerals and vitamins. Fibre was also important: herbivores could digest it, omnivores and carnivores could not, but all three needed it. Milk was the perfect diet for new-borns but low in fibre for more mature animals, so could only be part of a balanced diet. A clean water supply was also vital. Excess nutrients may also be a problem exemplified by obesity and excess of non-water-soluble vitamins. Excess water-soluble B vitamins are not possible as they cannot build up and are excreted in the urine.

Housing, shelter and accommodation were also important: too hot or too cold for that species was bad, air change was good as reduced the chance of airborne infection. On the other hand, chilling by high-level cold air change may not be good. The same with cleanliness and hygiene reducing surface infection. All these are logical preventive measures but since Edward Jenner's work with smallpox, nothing has prevented more death and disease in humans and animals than vaccination. The principle is simple in that a piece of the infective agent or a modified or dead version of the infected agent is introduced to the patient who is not suffering from the disease and later develops resistance or immunity. That immune response can be either an antibody reaction or a so-called cell immune response or a mixture of both. As a result, the human or animal has increased resistance to a disease it has never actually met or improved resistance to a disease it has long since forgotten.

There is a virus that causes vesicles or viral blisters on cow's teats called cowpox; it is caused by a pox virus called Vaccinia. Jenner had noticed that milkmaids had lovely skin and were never disfigured by the ravages of smallpox. He correctly assumed this might be due to the girls having contact with Vaccinia or cowpox. He then proved if the liquid from a cowpox vesicle was scratched on the skin, protection against smallpox was obtained.

Hence the term "vaccination". Cowpox, the harmless disease of cattle, and smallpox, the ravaging illness with 30% death rate of humans, are closely related viruses: both are *Variola* viruses and if humans exposed to the former *Variola vaccinia* they are protected against *Variola major* and the similar *Variola minor*.

As the exams approached, we all started to worry about getting a job after we qualified. I was spending the odd weekend in the Gloucestershire village of Berkeley, the very village where Edward Jenner had done his work on smallpox in 1798 and visited a local practice in Wotton-under-Edge owned by a year mate's father. When I visited, he offered me a job and I accepted as I knew there were no vacancies at my foster practice. He was short of a vet and wanted me to start as soon as possible, preferably the first of April. So that was the job sorted, back to studying.

Nerves were beginning to get the better of some of us. Previously extrovert characters were locking themselves in their studies, barely emerging for meals; others became similarly out of character by knocking at my door at 8.30 in the evening inviting me to the pub. I suppose I was a little out of character not going any evening until 10pm with just time for a single beer. This also helped the finances.

Before the exam proper was the Prize Examination Day. This was held on 7th March 1973 during the most important month of my life. There was a three-hour morning paper consisting of twenty tough questions, then an even tougher afternoon paper also of three hours with two questions needing answering out of an extremely limited choice. I had no intention or chance of winning a prize but with just five days until the third BVetMed medicine and seven days until the fourth BVetMed surgery written papers began it certainly focused me on my weaknesses.

The first preventive medicine paper was on 12th March and my heart sank: not a canine or feline question in sight but some poultry. The afternoon paper was better and only included horse, dog and cat medical problems. The third paper on the Tuesday seemed straightforward so the three hours quickly went by leaving three surgery papers for the rest of the week. The week flashed by with me finding plenty to say in the exam and after, but it remained to be seen how I had done. The following two weeks were full of practical exams and vivas and on the Friday afternoon the pass list was published. Forty-seven of us had passed out of fifty-seven, John August with honours in all subjects and he is now a Professor of Feline Medicine in Texas. I was saddened to be stood alongside one of the unfortunate candidates as he scanned up and down the results notice looking for his name and it certainly took the edge of my immediate personal celebration.

That afternoon I rang the Royal College for special permission to start practising immediately as I was worse than broke, I was busted.

They reluctantly gave me permission to start work on 1st April provided I promised to attend the induction ceremony at the RVC on the 10th April.

13

GLOUCESTERSHIRE

I started work on Monday 2nd April, 1973. It was a landmark day for the country. Not because I had started my veterinary career but because that was the first working day after Purchase Tax was replaced by Value Added Tax (VAT). Veterinary fees had not been taxed up until that day – well in fact the Sunday before. It was a great day to start work as everyone was so confused by the new tax that nobody questioned the young vet who had just seen them and were more confused by the tax of 10% added to their bill.

The induction day went well, and I was supervised by an immensely helpful colleague all day but slipped nicely below the radar thanks to the chancellor's VAT. The practice was very switched on as far as farm work was concerned but for dogs and cats was a little primitive. All surgery on these disadvantaged species was carried out using long-acting barbiturates and it was expected for all the neuters to sleep the day away.

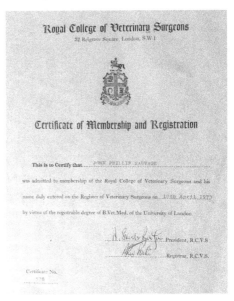

Certificate of membership and registration of the Royal College of Veterinary Surgeons – 1973

I was dreading my operating day on the Wednesday but first I had to cope with an evening surgery at one of the branches on the Tuesday night. I was faced with a little terrier with urinary problems so phoned the main practice and got hold of the vet who had been so helpful the day before. I described my problem and he advised me to get a urine sample. "There's a catheter in the drawer of the desk," he advised me. "Have you catheterised before?" he asked. I said yes and thanked him for his help. I had only catheterised male dogs and this was a fairly fat bitch. I asked her owner to hold this wonderfully behaved dog. The catheter passed first time and I got a very bloody urine sample easily. I then gave her a course of penicillin tablets and said I would get the sample analysed.

The next morning, I arrived in the practice saying to my colleague that I had got the sample from the six-year-old terrier bitch: were we going to send it to the lab or look at it with our own microscope? His jaw dropped. "I thought you said it was a dog?" he asked. I replied, "Yes, it is a dog but a female one."

"How on earth did you manage to catheterise a bitch at a branch surgery without sedation?" I just shrugged as if I had done it a hundred times. Had I been honest I would have told him I had never done it before, and if you ask me now, I have not done it since without sedation. The sample was sent to the lab and it was just a bacterial cystitis that responded well to my antibiotic course. Good job it did not need re-sampling. My operating day went well and after my catheterisation skill had been demonstrated I was left alone. I hit the veins OK and since the dogs and cats slept so long and so deeply no one noticed how long a dog castration, a couple of cat castrations and a cat spay had taken me.

The confusing VAT protected me from clinical questioning for the following six months as it surprisingly changed very quickly, going down to 8% which then made the calculation more difficult in those pre computer days, especially as many goods and petrol were 12.5%.

VAT issues did not rescue me on the farms, however, but I very quickly learned to respect the farmers' opinion and listen closely to what they told me. I clearly remember a pedigree Guernsey cow at peak lactation. Her temperature was normal, she was eating, she was grazing, milking very well with the spring flush of milk, she had calved three months previously, was not bulling and a full examination had revealed nothing. I had checked for a displaced stomach, checked for ketosis and mastitis. I was never good with the pear drop smell of ketosis but had dip tested her milk for the tell-tale of this metabolic problem that drives cows to burn fat in a diabetic way. But no ketones. Similarly, both the farmer and I had checked her udder and her milk for signs of mastitis but neither of us had found any sign.

He said again, "Not sure what but something is wrong." I trusted him so repeated my complete physical, everything normal, so with the medical message ringing in my ears, "Common things occur commonly," I checked her udder for the third time. The farmer had already checked three times so this was the sixth udder examination between the two of us. Three of the quarters were again clear as I squirted her milk on my boot and into my hands. Then on the last quarter there they were: tell-tale clots in her milk from the front left quarter. She did have early mastitis and immediate treatment of that quarter with an antibiotic tube and a four-day course of antibiotic reinforced my attitude of always listen to the herdsman – a message I took back to my colleagues at the induction from Mr Steele-Bodger as mentioned in the introduction.

The trip down the M4 that month for my RCVS induction went well and many of us met in the College Arms, a refurbished pub opposite the college, for a final drink before heading off to our jobs, wherever they were.

The next morning I was back at the practice and because of my weekday off, that month had to work two weekends during the height of the lambing season. The owner of the practice shared night duty with me meaning I did all the calls he thought I was up to and accompanying him to any he felt I was not up to. It was great because he knew his farmers well and knew where the easy lambing and calvings would be and where the tricky ones were.

He was also a stickler for making sure the mothers, whether calving or lambing, were suitably caught and restrained before we got there and as the farmers were never told who was coming – him with me or me alone – there was always a bucket of warm water, soap and towel waiting.

I learnt so much so quickly during that lambing and calving season, as my head was no sooner back on the pillow than I was woken by the next call. I very quickly managed the single lambs or calves with a malpositioned head that needed the head pushed back after getting the head rope on. It was hard physical work with cattle sometimes needing an epidural but the same technique with sheep requiring the ewe to be upturned to push the lamb's head back and needing dexterous fingers to organise the classic diving position necessary for normal forward birth. The legs also needed roping. Similarly, with multiple births, which leg belongs to which lamb is great training for the same scenario on a much larger, more physical scale of cattle obstetrics. Posterior presentations, where the calf or lamb is presented backwards, are usually easier as there is no head to get in the way; it is just a question of getting two back legs, from the same calf or lamb, in front of the correct backside and pulling the near new-born downwards. All this was manageable providing the imminent birth was recognised by the farmer but that was not always the case and a dead, dried-up calf or lamb was a tough call to salvage a live mother.

One of the cattle techniques I picked up was cattle blood transfusion. This was used mainly for cattle suffering from redwater, a tick-borne disease caused by protozoan parasite called *Babesia*. It causes the rupture of red blood cells and severe anaemia. I assisted the owner of the practice doing a couple of transfusion cases. Then a short time later I was on a farm testing and one of the cows was down in the yard where she collapsed before milking; although pale it was not redwater. She had ruptured her milk vein in front of her udder trying to jump a gate. The haemorrhage was just under the skin, but the blood loss was so substantial I had to transfuse her. This involves bleeding a donor non-milker using a large needle into the jugular with blood running into a bottle with anticoagulant; the donor behaved perfectly and the collapsed cow responded well to the transfusion once I had managed to get a needle into her collapsed vein, but at least she sat still in the yard whilst I did the transfusion. At least, no need to worry about blood typing with the first cattle transfusion.

One of my roles in the practice was looking after the prison farm at HMP Leyhill, which is an open prison. One of my regular jobs was disbudding calves. This process involves injecting local anaesthetic to numb the local horn nerves, then applying a red hot Calor-heated specialised poker with a concave tip to burn out the young calves' horn buds so no horns grow. The procedure is a two-person job where mutual trust is important. The assistant holds the calf's jaw and one ear leaning the calf over his thigh with the calf's backside firmly in a corner. The disbudder then burns out the calf's horn bud but the hot iron is inches from both handlers and a fraction from the calf's eye.

I had got to know the prisoner who looked after the young stock well over several months and we were a good team. I had been told that in the open prison the majority of offenders were short-time prisoners in for crimes such as fraud. My timing asking my teammate what offence he had committed was to say the least bad. I had just placed the red-hot iron on the horn bud when I asked. "I killed my wife and daughter," he answered. I was so shocked that the iron slipped upwards, only just missing our faces. He went on to explain how it was due to a specific set of circumstances and he had been assessed low risk. Somehow, I managed to get through the morning but from then on I never asked a prisoner his offence. Lesson learnt.

As far as leisure activity went, I was invited by a neighbour to go gliding with him as he was a member at Bristol and Gloucester Gliding Club and had a share in a glider. He promised me after our tow up from a winch we would probably get one circuit and then land, but just my luck we hit the biggest thermal of that summer and up and up we went. It was a very strange experience to be so high without an engine and overall did nothing to cure me of my fear of flying: I was so pleased to get my feet on the ground again. I certainly did not want to take it up as a hobby and that was my one and only attempt to find a hobby during my time there and the extensive duty rota put paid to any others, including football refereeing.

In fact, I had learnt so much in my first six months in practice, especially about farm work at a time when calf prices were high and it was affordable to farmers for calves with severe diarrhoea to have life-saving veterinary attention including IV fluids and the newly introduced oral electrolytes. Nonetheless, because of the low standard of dog and cat care in the practice at the time, I was so pleased to get a call from my foster practice that a vacancy had arisen, and I could join them within the month as Stuart had given notice there.

14

MAIDSTONE

Within a month of being offered the job I was working in my dream practice. It was a lovely high-quality mix of work. Top quality equine work, high standard dog and cat cases and good standard cattle and sheep clients with even the odd pig farm. The perfect blend and even a reasonable amount of back garden poultry

It was a bird that caused my greatest embarrassment in front of a client. I was attending to a beautifully spoken lady with a powder-puff white miniature poodle and although she usually had house calls decided to come into a busy evening surgery when both consult rooms were in use. I had seen from the appointment book that one of us had to see a parrot from the local pub. I was so pleased as after its health check and vaccination I had been asked to clip the poodle's nails, and I heard the parrot called in next door. The poodle had looked at me in a funny way – a mixture of fear but trust – as I clipped her nails and then Janet came in to borrow the nail clippers as the parrot's beak and nails needed trimming. She greeted my client and went back next door.

The parrot had not vocalised or screeched to let my client know it was next door until Janet approached it and the bird shouted in a most human voice, "Sod off." I smiled at my client who was unaware it was a parrot next door and tried to explain but the best thing I could do was escort her out and go and help Janet. The language got worse and the waiting room was full. Angry parrots can be quite dangerous, and this was a big Amazon. I went to the x-ray room and grabbed the lead gauntlets and a big towel. "Sod off," the bird repeated as the pub landlady put the towel over his head and I grabbed his head from behind using my forefinger and thumb around his head, his neck in the palm of my hand and the rest of him wrapped in the towel with the landlady trying to avoid his emerging talons. "Sod off you bugger," he yelled. "F★★★ you," as Janet uncovered the towel enough for his beak to emerge and its overgrown hooked beak to be clipped. His nails were easier and the obscene language more muffled, but we succeeded.

The landlady apologised to the waiting room as she left saying she did not allow bad language in her pub, but her husband must have trained the bird when she was not present. I for one did not believe her and it was a highlight to take friends to the pub where the beautiful parrot painted the air blue. Luckily, the bird was given a private appointment whenever the procedure needed repeating and each time he had more colourful vocabulary.

In March 1974 it was time was to collect my degree from the Chancellor of the University of London at the Royal Albert Hall. The Batchelor of Veterinary Medicine degree meant hiring a gown: it was a distinctive purple colour and I was proud to walk out when my name was called, and I was presented with my degree by none other than Queen Elizabeth the Queen Mother who was then Chancellor of the University. I was proud and smiling but not as proud as my mother who attended the ceremony and told me afterwards my smile with my big dimples was so broad that after shaking my hand the great lady's gaze followed me off the stage. Well, that's my mother's version of events so who am I to argue with her? I owed her so much for encouraging me to get those O levels, then A levels, then at last my veterinary degree. The fact my father never quite managed to give me my grant money was forgotten, and although he was at work that afternoon did not mean that he too was not proud of me. They both sacrificed for me and not once suggested I leave school and get a real job, abandoning my crazy dream of being a vet.

The duty rota was less frequent than Gloucestershire, just one weekend in three and one night duty a week. On one of the calls there was a seven-year-old chestnut hunter gelding with a fresh barbed wire cut about an inch above the hoof. The first thing to do was scissor clip the hair from around the wound and cleanse it. The laceration was not particularly ripped as is usual with barbed wire but was a deep cut running half way around the foot. I stitched it under local anaesthetic after freshening the wound and then sprayed the wound with antiseptic spray, remembering to give anti-tetanus and antibiotic. Two days later it was healing well, and AC called me back as I said good morning to him, grunting at me that it was not usual to stitch anything below the fetlock; but I seemed to have gotten away with it thanks to the big bites of the stitches, meaning the suture needle penetration was quite a distance from the wound. Two weeks later he told me he had removed the sutures and that I would make a reasonable equine surgeon, but I do not think he ever forgave me for taking his parking space or pranging his car.

An extremely useful techno tool for practices before phone pagers and mobile phones was short-wave radio. These were invaluable when out on calls and mine came in very handy one day when heading across Maidstone. I was in traffic near the centre of town when I heard screaming. It was so ear piercing I thought it was more than one voice but then realised it was a woman howling at the top of her voice. I got straight on the radio asking for the receptionist to contact emergency services, suspecting a terrorist attack. She rang them and then told me that all services were aware of an incident in the middle of Maidstone.

So, I parked my car and walked ten yards towards the screaming and realised it was near a bus parked at a bus stop. I rushed around the front of a bus and just in front of the entry door was a woman lying near the kerb yelling with the bus stationary with its front wheel on her foot. The driver had obviously run over an over-enthusiastic passenger trying to board at the stop and instead of moving the bus off her foot, with all the screaming was now frozen, half in half out of his cab. So afraid of making the situation worse he was making it worse. I yelled at him to get in the cab and move the bus. "Forward or back?" he asked. As the full weight was on the foot I shouted back, "Either but move now." He did as I said, driving forward, and immediately the screaming stopped. The lady seemed to be in her forties and was wearing robust shoes.

As she lay there, she asked me, "Will I lose my foot? Are you a doctor?" I replied, "I am a vet, and your foot will be fine." She did not seem reassured and asked the same question again. I stopped anyone taking the shoe off. Then an ambulance came and took her away. I rang the hospital twice to find out how she was but as I did not know her name and was not a relative, they would not give me any information and since nothing appeared in the local paper "no news was good news", or so I hoped.

Janet was an excellent surgeon and as well as me the practice had just taken on a husband-and-wife team of vets. One day I was consulting, and Janet and one of the new vets were operating on a bitch with pyometra, a womb infection. I had performed my first hysterectomy treatment of a case the month before but in this one the womb ruptured during surgery and they wanted to get permission from the client for the dog to be put to sleep without being allowed to wake from the anaesthetic as they felt peritonitis was inevitable. I argued that surely the abdomen could be flushed with saline once the ruptured womb was removed and the dog stood a chance of recovery with strong antibiotic use. It is a Roman saying that "Where there is life there is hope." I was overruled, and permission was obtained and the dog put to sleep. This was 1974 and twenty years later I had a similar case, and it did survive but perhaps antibiotics were stronger by then and no two cases are the same?

This was the year of the three-day week and the miners' strike. The TV stations had to close down at 10.30pm and there were a lot of power cuts. I was living in the same flat over the surgery that I had stayed in as a student guest of Stuart and most evenings were candlelit at some stage during the winter of 1974; I often just went to bed at 10.30.

During a night of that "Winter of Discontent" I was woken as I heard footsteps down my flat corridor and then a knock on my bedroom door. It was a policeman waking me up to tell me the river had burst its banks and Maidstone was flooding. I got out of bed and looked out of my bedroom window overlooking Earl Street and could see the floodwater in the moonlight nearly up to Museum Street. Luckily, the practice did not flood but it did re-locate that summer to a big house on nearby Holland Road. It was a purpose-built conversion and a great place to practise.

I also bought a little terraced cottage that summer near the village of Sutton Valence, I think for £14,000. I had to struggle to raise the deposit but by then I had paid back my overdraft acquired as a student and obtained a mortgage for £10,000 from a building society. I went to see a local bank manager who argued I could not afford to buy a house. House prices will never go up again like they did in the sixties, he said, and the rate on a house would make it unaffordable. I showed him that since the cottage was rural, not on mains drainage and did not have streetlights, the rates were low. He turned me down on the £400 I was short of the deposit. I was determined to buy the house and drew cash on my Barclaycard to pay the deposit. Then, like now, I knew not to borrow on a credit card as the interest rate was so high, especially for a cash withdrawal. No easy APR figures given then, but I knew it was high.

I went ahead and bought the house and very quickly paid off the credit card as inflation hit double figures and house prices rocketed. The rapid increase in the value of my house proved the bank manager wrong and they were meant to know about these things.

One evening I was asked to help at the local RSPCA clinic in Maidstone. The local practices supported the charity by manning the clinic regularly when no RSPCA vet was available. The clinic was going well and remarkably busy. It was quite enjoyable consulting without any pressure to charge fees or, worse, justify fees. Many of the pet owners were just so grateful for the help with pets they really could not afford.

There was one lovely ten-year-old mongrel with several massive ulcerative mammary tumours running in a chain along the underside of her body. I discussed the option of radical surgery and called in the RSPCA inspector who was there at the time. He said the nearest operating facility was the Harmsworth in London, but the owner decided to decline the surgical route and made the tough but inevitable decision to have the dog "put to sleep". The owner did not to stay as I drew up the barbiturates into a syringe, at which point the inspector offered to do it. The waiting room was full, so I accepted his offer, holding out the half-prepared lethal dose.

"I will be fine," he said and took the dog but not the drug. I wrongly assumed that he had a dose prepared elsewhere and had been trained at IV. Half way through the next consultation there was a loud bang of a gunshot. I was shocked, as was the lady I was talking to. The little bitch's owner had thankfully already rushed home. I charged out of the room into the yard at the back. The inspector was standing over the dead dog with a revolver in his hand. He saw my shock and said, "I always do the humane killing." I was stunned and made sure that if any of our vets did the clinic in future, they would carry out their own euthanasias. Can you imagine an RSPCA inspector behaving like that now?

As well as the new bright veterinary facilities in the house at the new practice, there was also a state-of-the-art equine operating theatre built in the gardens.

On one of my night duties, I was called to a horse that had staked itself up between its left foreleg and its chest. When people say a horse is bleeding badly, I usually find the cut horse has stopped bleeding by the time I arrive, usually within 20 minutes to an emergency, and they have exaggerated the blood loss. A little blood goes a long way. I arrived at the stable and there was the horse. The owner's hands were covered in blood and blood dripping as he stood with a cloth pressed up in the wound. He was reluctant to take his hand away to show me but when he did blood literally gushed out the wound. I put my cleansed right hand in the wound, and it went in up to the forearm, but blood rushed around me and onto the stable floor. The only thing I had nearby was a roll of cotton wool, so I pushed this in the hole and noticed if we positioned the horse's leg inwards, the leg itself with the cotton wools helped stop the haemorrhage.

We alerted the practice and got the hunter into a horse box and the owner and I got the patient to the equine theatre where everyone including RJ and two other vets were waiting. Sadly, the horse lost more blood as they wanted the leg position changed and removed my cotton wool roll. The blood gushed and my roll quickly replaced with another. The horse was anaesthetised and lying on its right flank stopped the gushing. Over the next hour the major arteries and veins that had been penetrated by the stake were tied off, or more accurately the major arteries and veins penetrated by the stake were partially tied off (ligated).

The blood leakage post-op was still tremendous, even if the wound was widened to locate the vessels it was still a small wound. Some of us argued to extend the wound and some to try and limit the extension. Having seen the gush originally, I belonged to the aggressive opening of the wound, but the more senior conservative opinion won out. The owners did not get to vote on this as they had been sent home with the horse box. Sadly, the horse died the next day; after recovery from the anaesthetic it stood, and blood again poured out of the sealed wound and the poor beast collapsed and died. I suspect it would have been a similar outcome if a more radical surgical approach had been taken as I suspect the severed artery and vein were too major for adequate ligation.

Little did I realise that one of the junior nurses that night would become my wife and the mother of my son, Ross.

1975 was a difficult year with the practice expanding rapidly with four new vets employed and several other new employees as well as the cost of the new premises: the economics both within the practice and nationally were not good. UK unemployment reached a million and was still rising and inflation reached 25%. I know the practice had the same bank manager and bank that refused my house purchase loan. So, I suspect the bank put pressure on the partners regarding the business loans. As my salary was the highest, it became me as the longest-serving non-partner asked to find another job – as employment laws were vastly different then than now. I was asked to work a month's notice but was so upset I left immediately on that Friday and went home, picked up the *Vet Record,* the veterinary journal for jobs, and by the Monday was doing locum work, meaning I could stay in the new home I loved. My dream job had disappeared, and I had to wake up.

15

LOCUM

The word locum is an abbreviation of the Latin "locum tenens", someone who temporarily fulfils the duties of another. It usually applies to a physician or clergyman but also applies to a veterinary surgeon.

The following Monday I found myself in Tom's practice in the East End of London with a branch surgery at Dagenham. My work accommodation was the flat over the Dagenham surgery. The work was 95% dogs and cats but there was a little horse work. I quickly settled in and when not on duty commuted by car to Sutton Valence and my peaceful little cottage in the country.

I was in the practice during Christmas and I had several calls on Christmas Day either to see cases at Dagenham or make house calls. One call was to a little Jack Russell and they wanted a house call so as not to disturb their Christmas, so I added it to my list. The first two were incredibly grateful for having house calls, offering drinks and hospitality which I declined, and then I got to the third. The door was just about opened by a teenager whilst mum and dad and the rest of a large family were sat around the dinner table not yet eating but drinking and chatting. "Hey, Mum the dog man is here," he shouted as I was pointed to a basket in the corner of the room and in it sat a shivering JRT lying on a little sheet. I asked questions about if she was vaccinated and the mother just leant over her shoulder and said "Yes." I asked "When?" "As a puppy," the father grunted from the table.

"How old is she? What's her name?"

"Ten, I think. Suzy," said the mother. I did not bother telling them that dogs need boosters. I took her temperature: it was high 103F

(39.4C) and tried to listen to her lungs and heart with my stethoscope but there was so much noise from the TV and the dining table I had to ask for quiet please but got no reply. I stood and raised my voice.

"Sorry to disturb your Christmas but this little dog is terribly ill. Please bring me a blanket, turn off the TV and be quiet for a minute so I can listen to her heart and lungs."

There was a hush at the table. The teenage boy who had let me in got up and turned down the exceptionally large TV a fraction, the mother fetched an old blanket and I listened to Suzy's wheezy little chest in the few moments' relative hush before the TV was switched up and the chatter began again. I injected Suzy and counted out some pills by her. I stood and walked to the table interrupting their conversation.

"Suzy has a high temperature and I think she has pneumonia. Please give her one antibiotic tablet three times a day and she may need to go into hospital." The family collectively acknowledged what I had said, then carried on with their Christmas chat as the mother impatiently got up to start serving their Christmas dinner. I saw myself out. My duty finished the Boxing Day morning and I set off from the flat for home after putting my little Christmas tree in the back of my car. Before I left, I checked Suzy's progress for the third time by ringing the owners. Different family members assured me she was much better and was taking her pills. Each time I rang I could hear the TV in the background but if she were eating and brighter, she did not need hospitalisation.

One day in the New Year I was called to a tinker's horse that was cut. The wound was too old to stitch so I was just going to clean it up to allow second intention (not skin to skin) healing, but it was a stallion and although he seemed calm when I examined him, as I lifted his rear right he kicked out. I had been trained how to pick up a horse's rear foot and it involves flexing the hoof whilst holding the Achilles tendon and getting close to the foot with my head, hopefully out of striking distance. Bang, he kicked me in the face, and I went flying out of the stable. I felt my eye socket was sore but after further attempts missing several kicks, I managed to clean and dress the wound and give anti-tetanus and antibiotic. That evening my left eye was black and blue. One of the clients in evening surgery joked, "Whose missus were you caught with then?" Nobody believed me that it was a horse kick. "Pull the other leg. No 'orses around here Guv." I simply said, "If I had pulled the stallion's leg a little better then he wouldn't have kicked me!"

Another equine call later in my first locum term there was from the police to destroy another horse hit by a car. When will drivers realise that when they encounter horses on roads, they are dealing with living unpredictable animals, not machines?

The dog and cat work at the practice was sophisticated and my boss Tom was a very skilled orthopaedic surgeon with all the specialist orthopaedic equipment we in the veterinary profession referred to as "toys".

Because it was a busy urban practice there was a sophisticated bone operation almost every afternoon as road traffic accident (RTA) cases were common and during my first month's locum there I assisted on many of these fracture repairs and if Tom was busy did some myself. Using pins in cats with fractured femurs was routine and I was soon clocking up several cases. In no time at all I was repairing similar fractures in dogs.

My month soon came to an end and I was due to do a week in a practice in Andover during the April of 1976. It was for a single-handed very well organised small animal practitioner with a well-trained following. He had obviously warned his clients he was away, and I only saw a couple of minor stitch-ups under local; there were no routine ops. He had given his receptionist and nurse the week off, so I saw a couple of minor digestive upsets in dogs on the medical side and the highlight of my week was watching Southampton win the FA cup on TV. When the owner returned at 9am on the Monday, the receptionist having been there from 7.30 booking appointments, I apologised for how quiet I had been. "That's what I hoped," he said as he wrote me a cheque for my locum fee.

While sitting around in Andover waiting for the phone to ring when it would not, I decided locuming was not my future: I would set up my own practice in Sutton Valence. There was a shop for sale there and I would set up my own "one-man-band". Being a sole practitioner was not my dream of being in a great partnership, but that had not gone well either. Over the next month or so while back locuming for Tom in the East End, I put in an offer on the shop depending on planning, and did some bottom-up accounting whilst in Andover and wrote a budget which I knew bank managers would require. By bottom-up accounting I mean decide what the profit needs to be, add that figure to the forecasted fixed and variable costs to forecast turnover. The turnover was then divided by a forecast average transaction fee to produce the number of transactions needed. Assuming each client uses the practice twice a year gives the number of clients. I had certainly done my homework in Andover.

Back at Tom's practice I had a couple of bad experiences. Firstly, having parked the car outside the practice in Ilford and going inside to collect the stock, five minutes later I went outside to load the stock and set off, but the car had gone. I went back inside assuming the nurses were playing one of their frequent jokes on me and asked who had moved my car with the spare keys, but they all kept very straight faces and looked blank. I held up my car keys and told them I had locked it outside. The police were very quickly at the practice asking if any drugs were in the car. I told them, "Enough penicillin to treat venereal disease in a herd of elephants." "Any strong controlled drugs?" they asked. "Two bottles of pethidine, a morphine type drug," I replied, thanking my lucky stars I had recently put the gun back in the safe after my recent night duty.

Within half an hour the car was found dumped in the docklands minus only the radio – with all the drugs in the boot. On returning it the police said the thieves must have heard on police radio about the car and quickly abandoned it as "too hot to handle".

My other bad memory occurred in the consulting room at Ilford. I was carrying out a routine puppy check and first vaccination. The clients were a tiny little lady and her massive body-built boyfriend. The puppy for just eight weeks old was already being extremely aggressive for a little Shetland Sheepdog and the petite lady was worried. As I examined him, he growled and tried to bite me, then his owner. I showed her how to gently hold the puppy in a circular two-handed way, a version of Mo Farah's heart-shape signal around the little chap's neck so he could not hurt either of us and that would not harm him. Next thing I was lifted with both my feet off the ground by the boyfriend, the puppy was under his left arm and the right was around my collar and I was half way up the wall. The girlfriend was tugging on his lifting arm as he said, "Don't yo' dare 'urt my lit'le puppy."

"Put him down," she ordered and suddenly my feet dropped to the floor as he decided she meant me and not the puppy. At that she sent the big man out of the room, leaving me to vaccinate the puppy with her and discuss aggressive behaviour in her household. Which seemed to be a common theme, but she was such a sweet lady I am sure she sorted them both out. I certainly hope so.

Around March 1976 I had applied to do a locum in Rotherham for later in the summer, but they requested an interview. I was going to the veterinary conference in London that Easter but nobody from the practice was going so one Friday I drove all the way to Rotherham and back for an interview. As I arrived about 11am all the nurses and receptionists were on a coffee break. I was called into the senior partner's office as he was brought a cup of coffee, but I quickly got the hint: I was not worthy of proper "Yorkshire hospitality". The interview was on the same level as the one at Cambridge, only more unpleasant. In the end I was offered two weeks' work the following August at below the going rate and sent off without any offer of payment for my day or mileage, let alone a cup of tea or coffee.

My plans for my own practice were going well. I had got planning permission and was beginning to sort out the purchase of the shop as by now I had enough equity in my cottage, when I saw an advertisement in the *Vet Record* from the Cranbrook practice. I decided to apply and was very quickly offered an interview. I was interviewed by two of the partners and whilst pleasant and sociable, had elements of what is now known as "good cop-bad cop" about it. Eric was kind, friendly and easy going but Doug was controversial, asking about my bitch spay technique and critical of not just my technique but the suture materials I said I would use. Then he asked me, "What do you regard as an emergency?" I safely replied, "Whatever the client and I decided in a telephone discussion was an emergency."

"So," he asked, "what if a client rings at one in the morning and wants her dog's anal glands emptied?"

I diplomatically replied, "If the owner felt the problem was urgent and happy to pay the out of hours' fee, I would certainly go."

At this point the third partner Larry arrived in the room. Larry took me off on a visit with him asking all sorts of questions about my plans, especially the setting up in Sutton Valence. He had obviously heard about my planning permission. He told me the practice only employed potential partners and what did I think. I said I did not think Doug liked me. "Nonsense," he said. "Doug is charming, and I know he likes you." I told him about the anal glands question, and he laughed.

"That's because somebody rang him the other night at one in the morning saying the dog was so uncomfortable would he go to do the anal glands and he refused to go saying it was not an emergency."

This was late July and the three of them said they needed to discuss things with a fourth partner on holiday that week and they would get back to me.

I told them I had a two-week locum in Rotherham booked for the first two weeks in August and gave them the practice number.

I set off for Rotherham on a Sunday, arriving at the flat in the small ex mining town of Maltby. I parked outside, collected the keys from a neighbour as arranged and went in. The downstairs was a typical branch surgery and the flat upstairs seemed to be covered in coal dust from before the last pit closed. This was not a major issue, but the lack of bedding was. I spent a chilly night under a cover with a cushion as a pillow. The next morning, I went to the main surgery and met Mr

A, a partner in the practice. The senior partner who had interviewed me was now too ill to practise. I asked for some bedding and he told me I should have brought some. I set about my day's work in what was now a 99% small animal practice.

That afternoon I was at the Maltby surgery before heading to Rotherham for the evening surgery. As I got in my car, I saw the parking ticket fluttering under my wipers. I drove to Rotherham and was quickly told by Mr A that locums always got parking tickets outside the surgery. When asked why he did not tell me I was greeted with, "Not my problem." At least that night when I got back to Maltby there was bedding at the flat. I spent the evening cleaning and missing my little cottage in Sutton Valence.

The next day I went to Rotherham for my operating day. I was not allowed into Mr A's operating theatre but as there were just three dental treatments, I did not need the theatre.

After my morning in the main branch the team seemed to melt, and I was offered a cup of tea after all my dental work which was pretty well just straightforward extractions of wobbly loose teeth.

That afternoon an emergency hysterectomy came in with a bitch with pyometra. She was an eight-year-old collie who had been in season and now was dripping pus from her vulva. She was very poorly and very thirsty. The nurses' faces dropped when I told them the bitch needed emergency surgery and I was told, "But Mr A is off and cannot be disturbed." "Let us not disturb him then," I said. "Get the theatre ready please." "But it's Mr A's theatre," I was told. I repeated my instructions and, as jaws dropped further, added I needed an IV drip for the patient.

We prepped the lovely dog, set up the drip and within the hour the dog was recovering minus a womb full of pus and two ovaries. The next day Mr A came up to me at the surgery and I was expecting a telling off for using his operating theatre, but he just told me he had discharged the collie and the owner was pleased.

That Wednesday night the phone rang and it was Doug from Cranbrook offering me the job. When I said I was surprised after the interview, he said he was just seeing how I responded under pressure. I said I would give him my answer within the week when I was home.

On my penultimate day at the Rotherham practice, Mr A called me to the x-ray viewer; on it was a lateral view of a dog's abdomen with what clearly looked like a stone lodged in the dog's gut. He told me he was thinking of operating but hoped the stone would pass. "What are the symptoms?" I asked and was told the history of an eleven-month-old puppy male GSD with intermittent vomiting and a palpable lump in the posterior abdomen. "When did he last vomit?"

He told me "that morning and nothing passed". I then examined the dog and we agreed on surgery that afternoon if there was any more vomiting, and for the second time during my stay an IV drip was prepared. That afternoon Mr A asked for his theatre to be prepared as the dog vomited again. He turned to me and said, "I will do the GA, you do the surgery." I found bowel clamps and extra swabs and followed Mr A into his theatre. The op went well, and no bowel needed resecting, just a small incision on some nice fresh intestine in front of the FB (foreign body) – by in front I mean further down the bowel, not in the bruised sore parts through which the stone had passed. The stone milked easily through the incision between the bowel clamps and I sutured the gut wall and then repaired the midline entry wound.

Afterwards, Mr A said so the nurse could hear him that the anaesthetic went well and that was such an important part of the procedure. I agreed and left his theatre. Later that afternoon he invited me to supper at his home and he and his wife were all sweetness and light, telling me they were building a house called "Gillymich" because his name was Michael and hers Gill! I said, "What a great name for a house." He then said I was just the sort of chap he was looking for as a partner as the senior partner was retiring. I replied I could not possibly consider that after the way he had treated me at the practice or with the outstanding parking ticket. I was finishing the next day and promised to let him know my answer. I walked into the Rotherham surgery and he went straight to the till, opening it and getting the exact parking fine out, although I had never told him the amount, and gave it to me. I told him I had another offer and I would give him my decision after the weekend. Later that afternoon I headed back home with the team waving me off in a very friendly manner. Too little too late, I thought as I drove off, but I had kept my options open.

I had a decision to make. Either set up my own practice and buy the shop in Sutton Valence, join the Cranbrook practice as an assistant or join the Rotherham practice as a partner. I made my decision and made the necessary phone calls. It was now the middle of August and I had a final one-week locum spell booked for Tom's practice in Ilford and I was again based in Dagenham. The car workers were on strike when I was doing an evening surgery and a little Yorkshire terrier bitch was presented. She was 12 years old, was in season the month before, was very thirsty and off her food. I thought she had a pyometra and explained to her owner, giving him the options. Ideally his little dog needed some blood tests to prove she just had pyometra alone and no other complications such as kidney or liver failure or concurrent diabetes. Her owner was a nice man in overalls and asked how much the test and surgery would be. I estimated £100. "That's a lot," he said. I agreed and said his little dog was incredibly old and terribly ill and surgery may not even work, so he could make a tough but perhaps kind decision to put her to sleep.

He wiped a tear from his eye and reached into his overall, pulling out some money. He counted out £25 saying could he pay this much immediately and, as soon as the strike was over, pay the rest. "Do you work at Fords?" I asked. "No," he said. "I am a window cleaner, and nobody wants me while the strike is on." I agreed to do the tests and operation the next day and it was an uncomplicated pyometra apart from also needing several tooth extractions and a clean and polish of her remaining teeth. The little dog made a fantastic recovery, and I heard the following week that the window cleaner paid a lump sum off his bill and a week later the strike was over and he paid it off in full.

But I had left to start at Cranbrook during the lovely September of 1976. I also got married that month.

16

CRANBROOK

The practice at Cranbrook was not as sophisticated a cattle practice as Gloucestershire, or a high-quality equine practice as Maidstone or as leading edge on small animal orthopaedics as Ilford but it was closely behind these and far ahead of Rotherham, which ironically was a registered hospital.

The other great thing about Cranbrook was the charm and care of the personalities in the practice. When I joined, I was the only assistant to the four partners and as I got to know them, I liked all four. The main reason they needed another vet was they had recently got a meat hygiene contract from the local borough council so that lamb meat could be exported to Europe. My presence released one of them every day for this certification duty.

It was a truly mixed practice in the picturesque Wealden town with branches in the commuter villages of Headcorn and Marden. Gloucestershire was pretty but Kent really is the "Garden of England". One of the cases I saw in the first week was another case of womb infection (pyometra), this time in an otherwise fit looking Black Labrador. She was certainly not fit on the day I saw her: there was a purulent mucky discharge, she was very thirsty and vomiting. It was a house call to a beautiful Wealden hall house characteristic of the area and not only of architectural value. As she was only seven, I was sure the owner would agree to an emergency hysterectomy. To my shock, this obviously wealthy owner of a bookshop in Staplehurst declined surgery and unlike the poor window cleaner said it was not financially viable. He could easily get another Labrador for shooting. I was so shocked I offered to do the operation and either re-home the dog or find some other solution. I got the impression that even if I had offered free surgery he would have declined.

I was looking for a solution when he insisted I put the lovely dog to sleep. I told him the cost of the visit, examination and euthanasia would come to more than some temporary treatment before an operation, but he was almost sadistically determined to have the dog put to sleep, threatening to shoot her if I did not "Immediately put her out of her misery". I reluctantly drew up the barbiturate and found an easy vein as she was so good and feeling so poorly that she just went straight off. I could hardly talk to her ex-owner after that, thinking of the great contrast between an animal lover – the window cleaner – and an animal user – the bookshop owner.

The bookshop owner was not a typical client and I enjoyed all aspects of the work with my day starting by consulting at one of the surgeries and finishing at another with visits in between. With five of us, each had one day a week operating. The work was varied, and I benefited so much from the experiences gained in my previous practices. Most of the clients including the farmers were charming and I was so pleased I had not set up my one-man practice in Sutton Valence.

My first weekend was in sole charge because everyone else in the practice was heading to the wedding of one of our part-time receptionists, a farmer's daughter Diana and her local solicitor husband Nick, who are now great friends as well as long-term clients. Our weekends were split then: two vets did Saturday morning, one stayed on duty all day Saturday and the other did Friday and Sunday. Doug finished at 12 so he could get to the wedding.

It was a normal Saturday, but all was quiet until I was called to a local riding stables where one of the horses was a bit stiff. Everything was normal on examination, except the seven-year-old gelding had what I can only describe as a slightly anxious facial expression and a slightly stiff action when trotted in the yard. I started to wonder if this was a case of tetanus and my suspicions were further raised when I lifted his head by pushing his chin and muzzle up. The third eyelid came immediately in front of his eyes and I remember Johnny G saying that was a classic sign of early tetanus before the muscle rigidity became obvious.

I asked if he was vaccinated and the riding school owners confirmed not. Tetanus and botulism are both examples of bacterial infections where the symptoms are caused by the bacterial toxin released, not the bacteria itself. I filled him with a massive dose of penicillin and tetanus antiserum and asked if one of my partners could check on him the next day. Doug confirmed my diagnosis and the gelding responded well to treatment as the disease had been caught early. Neither of us found a primary wound but not all cases have one. All the horses in the stables were then vaccinated: another example of prevention being better than cure for the rest but after the horse had bolted for the individual gelding.

Years later I was called by a farmer Ned who ran the local pheasant shoot. He was losing birds by the dozen at all ages. I suspected some toxic rather than infectious cause, but tests proved it was botulism where the bacterium releases the toxin which causes paralysis and death, so it was both an infection and a toxic poisoning. It was suspected that ducks from his pond had started the infection and spread it to the pheasants. The pheasants were temporarily moved away, and the deaths stopped.

There was one lady farmer client who had a tough reputation and would not let one of the partners on her farm after a calving had not gone well. Then the dreaded night-duty phone call came. It was Morri and she did not want me to go to her calving Hereford cow, telling the duty nurse to contact Larry. I told her Larry was not available and I would get straight there.

"The head is back," she said, "and that's how the last calf died." I reassured her I would try to help.

Twenty minutes later on the farm, the first job was to catch the cow. No farmers seemed as well trained as in Gloucestershire where the cow was already tethered and the bucket of hot water standing by. Eventually the cow was caught and tethered and later still the bucket of not-so-warm water. I cleansed my hands and arms, wearing the same type of parturition gown I wore for the yard of ale during freshers' week. On the internal vaginal examination, I could feel two front legs belonging to the same calf and no head. I put a rope on each then reached in to find the head. The cow was exhausted so I was easily able to push the legs back a little and I felt one of the legs pull back. I reached in again and felt the head turned back. By chance I poked the poor calf in the eye. It seemed to shake its head and as its front feet had been pushed back went into the normal dive position. I quickly put on the head rope behind the ears and pulled all three ropes. The cow responded and started straining again and soon with a rush of bloody fluid a red-and-white Hereford bull calf came into the world.

Morri was impressed and we stayed friends. I was so lucky with that first calving, but it did give me credence for later at the farm and with her dogs if things did not go so well.

One of the farm clients who followed me from the Maidstone practice to Cranbrook was Nick. He farmed in Sutton Valence with a beautiful pedigree Sussex herd. He always had local friends to help him and originally his father managed his two local farms. At first it was Chris who helped him before he pursued his career as a hotelier, followed by Simon before he pursued his as a publisher. I always enjoyed the banter during my visits to the farms although I was usually the target for their slightly sarcastic form of humour. Nonetheless, the hours spent doing routine cattle work was enjoyable, come rain or shine, and the odd invitation in the magnificent farmhouse for a game of snooker which I usually lost was memorable.

My first three months in the practice flashed by and it was Christmas in no time. The partners showed me their appreciation by giving me a handsome Christmas bonus. The duties were evenly shared, and Larry stressed again as he gave me the bonus that almost all assistants in the practice became partners. I again mentioned my willingness to buy in but needed to see the practice books and know the costs. Larry also asked if I would go on the Local Veterinary Inspector (LVI) course and meat hygiene course, the former to TB and brucellosis test cattle as well as dog and cat export certification if owners moved abroad or sold puppies abroad, and the latter to certify meat for export. The LVI course was in Maidstone and the Ministry vet was keen to discuss how badgers in the area were known to carry TB. That was at the beginning of my veterinary career; now at the end of it the debate still goes on. I did TB and brucellosis blood tests under supervision and was awarded my LVI.

My first few brucellosis blood tests went well and then two went horribly wrong: at the first, cattle got out of their pen and dented my new practice car; at the second, I had just finished blood testing Hugh Richards' herd of 200 Friesian dairy cows in Biddenden when walking back to the car I dropped the box and out of the 200 samples about 70 bottles had broken. This meant going through the whole herd selecting the cows I needed and resampling them which took about another two hours. Luckily, I did not have to go back to Cranbrook for more sample bottles and Hugh saw the funny side of it saying that even with the delay we were quicker than some Ministry vets had been who did his last test.

I then had to go to an abattoir in Cardiff to obtain my LVI Meat. It was an interesting course, but I was shocked to see kosher slaughter techniques. This sadly involved a revolving crush that allowed the rabbi easy access to cut the beast's throat without any stunning. Again, this debate still carries on at the end of my career, but I must say the animals did not seem to suffer apart from momentary disorientation, but halal and kosher slaughter does seem a harsh religious tradition.

When I got back from Cardiff, I could do my day a week at the sheep slaughterhouse in Lamberhurst and I found that process humane, unless again the halal process was used which did not allow stunning. Nothing I have seen would turn me vegetarian or vegan as I think farms without livestock are dead, desolate places and the human experience would be poorer without our farm animal population – but perhaps we should continue to review our animal welfare standards.

Late one evening I was called to a pedigree Shetland foaling by a long-standing client of the practice just over the border in East Sussex. Foalings can have similar complications to calvings and lambings but since labour is much shorter and more intense and violent, things can go horribly wrong very quickly. The relatively longer neck and limbs of a foal make correction of presentation more hazardous and difficult. As it is such a short, sharp, dramatic private process, many who work all their lives with breeding horses may not witness the event. At the RVC we had an observation stable – a stable with an observation room attached and one-way glass – so the patient could be observed a bit like a John Le Carré version of George Orwell's "Animal Farm" and "1984". As a final year we collectively spent many hours there hoping to see a normal foaling but not one of us did.

Amanda, one of the nurses at Cranbrook, was not on duty that night so was free to leave the building and accompany me to Bodiam and assist me. The pony was on the ground thrashing and straining with one of the foal's hooves showing. An internal examination showed one of the forelegs was flexed backwards, preventing the normal dive into the world. As I was down struggling, Lady J asked in her beautiful and perfect aristocratic version of English, "Have you done many foalings?" To which I promptly replied as if offended, "I hope you are asking the nurse." This forced Amanda to reply "No."

Because the poor little mare was tired from her forceful unproductive straining, I managed to briefly push the whole foal back a fraction and straighten the flexed fetlock that was causing a jamming in the pelvic canal. Immediately, before I had a chance to put ropes on, the clever little mare pushed with all her strength and the lovely tiny little creature rushed into our presence. I had managed to correct birth malpresentations of dead foals in horses in my career so far, but it was a memorable evening because it was in fact my first of many live foalings.

In the summer of 1978 my partner, Larry, had been treating a young filly with colic. He had been to see it several times in the day and during evening surgery got another call from Anne, the owner. He asked me to go and see it again as I was on duty. He was particularly pessimistic about the case, telling me to take the gun with me as apparently the poor horse was down and unable to get up. I got to the field where the horse was kept next to the pub owned by Anne and her husband Ian. He was waiting by the field gate to a large orchard. I took some drugs I thought I might need and hopped over the gate and about 100 yards away there was the little filly lying flat out and looking distressed. She was breathing heavily and alarmingly there were no gut sounds.

An internal examination did nothing to convince me the horse would survive. I told Ian that both Larry and I thought she should be destroyed. He reluctantly agreed but said to go and tell his wife first. I had to go back to get the gun from the car so offered to go to the accommodation over the pub and tell Anne what needed doing. Before I went I injected some pain killer and some heart stimulant. At the doorway I could not make myself heard over the sound of a hoover. I went in and up the stairs: there was Anne hoovering like mad around their lounge. She told me it was to take her mind off the filly's plight. I obtained permission to shoot the horse and went back to the car to get the gun and a torch as the light was fading fast. Ian was back at the gate and we climbed over and went back to where the filly was, but she had gone. It took a half hour wandering in the dark orchard before we found her grazing normally. "Wonderful stuff you gave her," said Ian. "She had been down all day." We went back and told Anne who was still spring cleaning with a vengeance and tears of sorrow turned to tears of joy.

I rang the next day and the filly was still doing well. A few weeks later I was called again to Anne and Ian's. This time their dog Sheba, a lovely German Shepherd dog, had fallen down the stairs from their lounge and could not get up. On examination she was very wobbly, but no bones broken. Her eyes were flicking, and I wondered if she had a bout of the balance problem called Vestibulitis, but Ian then found all the pub's beer slop trays had been emptied and he suspected Sheba had drunk them dry. She also had very beery smelling breath.

Sheba was just drunk and was fine the next day after some non-steroidal anti-inflammatory tablets (NSAIDs). My two visits got me enough credence to be invited to Anne and Ian's Christmas morning drinks party every year from then on.

The following year was remarkably stimulating in mixed practice, but my interest slowly returned to the dogs and cats.

When I was at college there were very few textbooks on feline medicine, and I had devoured them. Although we were in a rural area there were plenty of catteries in the practice area, so I started to gather them and the cat breeders as clients. Canine medicine and surgery also held my interest so apart from the duties I began doing more and more routine small animal work and less and less large animal and equine work, although I did enough to keep my competence level up.

A year had gone by and little more was said about a partnership but then Eric asked me if I wanted to buy his house by the Marden surgery. The price was good so I agreed and again I was told a partnership deal would be on the table soon. Another year went by without the offer although I bought the house.

My son Ross was born on 8th May 1978, which was the thirty-third anniversary of VE Day. Interesting that I was born on Battle of Britain Day and him on Victory in Europe Day.

I have told the story of how I was kicked by the tinker's horse, but the most dangerous kick was one that missed. I was called to a yearling colt with colic and when I arrived he was lying flat out in the stable, sweat running off his body. His head was farthest from me and I could see his eyes rolling with pain. I walked in and pulled the stable door behind me but did not close it. In an instant, quicker than a cobra strike, he jumped up on his forelegs and lashed with both back legs. There was a loud bang as the hooves smashed into the stable door to my right and my left. The door flew open and in an instant he was down rolling in agony. An inch either side and I think I would have spent my life in a wheelchair. I quickly administered a massive dose of painkillers IV into his jugular while his neck was stretching with the pain. The relief was instantaneous and his owner who was lucky to be out of the way of the stable door flying open told me he was usually very well behaved and asked what I had given him. I told him pethidine and as the colt relaxed and stood up, I examined him. His gut was rumbling and gurgling very clearly on stethoscope examination and I diagnosed "spasmodic colic" and also then injected a spasmolytic drug. The colt made a great recovery, but I will never forget my experience of the hooves whistling past either side of my waist.

A few weeks later I was called to another colic case, this time belonging to a local GP doctor. On the telephone he was in a panic as he knew the treatment for colic was often pethidine and had administered some. Because the pony was now sweating, he was convinced he had overdosed it. I arrived at the doctor's house and was taken to the back where the pony was being walked to stop it rolling. It also had all the symptoms of spasmodic colic. The doctor said, "Have I overdosed him with pethidine?" I asked, "How much did you give?" "1ml," he replied and showed me the bottle. "I will give him another 12ml of the same strength as well as a spasmolytic," I told him, and he was genuinely shocked but also relieved that the underdose had caused no harm. I probably did not need to tell him that he should not administer a controlled or any other drug to his animals as I was certain he knew he had broken the law. "It is OK for me to treat humans with their agreement, not that I would, but against the rules for you to treat animals!"

As my joining the partnership was still not finalised, I began to dream of African skies again as that continent had got into my blood, so I asked if all my annual holiday could be taken at once so I could go to South Africa with a dual-purpose view of a holiday and locum in a practice in Johannesburg, with a view to accepting a partnership out there unless a deal appeared on the table as Larry's line of no assistants, only partners, was wearing a little thin.

This certainly galvanised them, but the poker game went on with the partners allowing a month's leave but no offer on the table.

17

JOHANNESBURG

So, in early January 1979 we flew to Johannesburg for a month. The practice was in the leafy suburb of Kempton Park where there seemed to be a church on the corner of every block and my work colleagues were great. They quickly accepted me, and all aspects of practice were the same except that every dog case was made more complex by the need to consider and rule in or out concurrent tick fever caused by a malarial-type parasite called *Babesia*. This was a parasite I had known in Gloucestershire as a cause of redwater but only on home shores in cattle.

It is diagnosed using blood smears so inevitably I was seeing all the usual UK canine medical problems but had to check this disease was not also present. On its own the disease can cause appetite depression, blood in urine, jaundice and anaemia but as I say was often part of a complex presentation. Treatment for *Babesia* involved anti-parasitic injections, supportive care and sometimes blood transfusions, but as usual preventive measures were better using regular tick control.

Apartheid was present but not immediately obvious to me – except that all the Africans had to have permits to be in white suburbs and were all assigned to local townships to live. Some of the guys who worked for the practice could stay in little outbuildings adjoining the practice and only went home to their township and families in the suburban shanty towns on their days off. Apartheid may not have been obvious to me, but racism was. The owner of the practice's favourite saying was, "From Cape to Cairo: they are all the same."

I argued with him that the African fellows who worked for him were brilliant with languages. The fact they spoke a couple of tribal languages as well as English and Afrikaans surely reflected equal intellect to his "white supremacist" views. I am no linguist so anyone who can speak more than their mother tongue has my total respect. He just scoffed at my view saying I would find out. In fact, I found his world view awful.

When carrying out anaesthesia with a windpipe tube, a so-called endotracheal (ET) tube, so many got chewed as the dogs and cats woke up because the African male nurses did not take them out in time. The boss said this was an example of how stupid they were. Within my short time there I proved it was just a lack of training as so few of the vets were using them during surgery.

During my time off I enjoyed the climate and the outdoor lifestyle. It was great to see the African night sky and feel the sun on my face during the day. One evening I was having a BBQ with the other vets when Jackson, one of the African nurses rang, he had been knocked of his pedal bike and run over in a white suburb and the ambulance would not pick him up. We drove and found him limping at the side of the road by his mangled bike. There was no question of taking him to the local white hospital, so we drove to the nearest township hospital. It was a weekday night, but casualty was crowded. Seeing our white faces, we were ushered straight through to the doctor who thought Jackson had no fracture but wanted an x-ray. We went to radiography, which was quieter than casualty. He was immediately seen by a lovely Danish radiographer who proved there were no fractures. We asked how she got to be working in the township, which gave a glimmer of hope for South Africa's future when she replied, "People are people, and we all need medical help." Jackson the nurse was back at work by the end of the week, limping and bruised but thankful for our help.

Whilst in South Africa we even went to my first drive-in movie. It was "Superman", starring Christopher Reeve. I am not a fan of the genre, but it was so novel to park alongside what looked like a pair of parking meters in the practice van I was using and wind down the two side windows for speakers to be hooked on the inside of the window from those meters. The giant screen lit up and it was a great experience with Ross asleep in the back of the van.

I also had the following weekend off so borrowed the van with the practice owner's permission and drove the four-and-a-half-hour trip to Kruger Park – 450km (280 miles). We stayed in a great safari lodge, but the game viewing was not as good as East Africa as the grass was long from the rainy season. Nonetheless I saw plenty of zebra and impala and a guide took us to see lion but as always, the view was brief because of the tall savannah grassland.

The weekend was over quickly and after a morning game drive it was time to head back to Johannesburg. All the other vets warned me that the owner of the practice would spend my last week encouraging me to join the practice and although I liked the practice I did not like his racist attitude or some of his clinical practices.

During an evening meal the question of my returning and payment for my locuming was discussed. He offered to pay me in Kruger Rands, those beautiful gold coins, as there were currency controls in place, and he said I could take them out in my luggage if I did not declare them. I said a cheque would be fine and told him my future was undecided regarding a partnership at home, but it did seem likely.

I had a contact in Barclays SA, an uncle of Graham, a farmer friend of mine. To get the cheque into the bank involved going into the city centre and all seemed very integrated; it was only at Barclays did I notice a "Whites Only" main door and a side door with a separate counter for "Non-Whites". I walked in the wrong door and told the teller I had an appointment with my friend's uncle, which caused a bit of a stir and I had to go round to the "whites only" door to gain access to the offices. For a small fee, my cheque was converted to pounds and deposited in my account. It seemed as far as the currency restrictions were concerned, it was a case of "who you knew".

We were soon on my flight from Johannesburg and the whole adventure had been self-financing, but I knew South Africa was too unstable to spend my veterinary career there, tempting though it was. On my return the discussions with Larry and the partners went on and it was agreed I would join the partnership on a junior basis the following year, April 1980, but had to sort out the finance myself in just over a year.

18

PREVENTION BETTER THAN CURE

In the spring and summer of 1979, a new disease struck the canine population. Ever since seeing practice I had seen cases of per-acute haemorrhagic gastro-enteritis or, in plain English, severe and sudden onset bloody vomiting and diarrhoea, thought to be caused by overgrowth of a strain of *E. coli bacteria* and a shock reaction to it toxins. The problem if untreated, and often when treated aggressively with IV fluids, oral rehydration fluids, antibiotic and sometimes corticosteroids for shock, could still be fatal. The new disease was equally difficult to treat but much more common.

We quickly found out from virology research groups that it was caused by a parvovirus. As well as causing the above symptoms in both adult dogs and puppies, it also caused cardiac damage and heart failure. We never saw the cardiac version, but the gastrointestinal version was extremely common, and the ward was full of dogs of all ages and sizes on drips. The mortality rate initially was exceedingly high, near 70%, but improved as clients spotted the disease earlier and we got more aggressive with therapy, especially IV fluids.

Within a month of the start of the canine parvovirus pandemic it was recognised that the cat parvovirus vaccine (panleucopaenia) gave some protection. My future partner Mel did all our drug purchasing and he secured a massive supply of the cat vaccine to use in our canine patients. All of us spent the next month vaccinating dogs with a cat vaccine and reminding clients of the other preventable diseases of dogs as they signed a consent form. There were no side effects.

Prevention really was better than cure. The cat vaccine seemed to work and slowly the number of intensive care dogs dropped and those who got the disease after cat vaccination seemed to get milder forms and zero mortality. Within six months dog vaccines included a parvovirus component and again Mel came up trumps, getting them first from New Zealand I seem to remember. Sadly, there are still cases of canine parvovirus as some members of the public have short memories of how important vaccines are.

So just as the practice was at its busiest, I was negotiating my buy in. I had to pay a price calculated on an average of the last three years' profits and they were flying in that last year due to parvovirus. It was like buying another house and about the same price. Thanks to the practice accountant and financial adviser David, I found one of the banks in Cranbrook high street willing to lend to me and started to sort my loan.

As the height of the parvovirus outbreak was calming, Mel and I went to Selhurst Park in London to watch Crystal Palace play Burnley. It was a Friday and at last we both had the weekend off. It was a vital game that if Palace won, they would be champions of Division 2 with guaranteed promotion to the top football league. It was the perfect opportunity to have a chat with Mel about the partnership. He was a keen Derby supporter and I was pleased to have a chance to chat one on one. What a fantastic night. The attendance was a record that still stands – 51,482 – and it would have been two less without us. Palace won 2-0 and it meant Palace joined Derby in the top division the next season. Mel seemed happy to have me as a business partner and I told him I had secured the finance.

I was looking forward to more football-friendly rivalry with Mel but within two years Mel left the partnership for personal reasons and I had to fill his role of drug purchaser and at the same time bought another tranche of practice equity, so now again there were four partners each having a 25% share.

Once Mel left the practice, I took over his role of drug and vaccine purchaser. I learnt a very harsh lesson very quickly when the ICI rep for Estrumate, a cattle hormone injection, came in and asked if I wanted the same order as Mel had the previous year. I agreed and some of the drug arrived. It was amazingly effective at bringing cows into season. It contained the drug called prostaglandin which my flatmate doing the extra year BSc had told me about. Here we were less than a decade later and it was one of the major cattle drugs, also useful for inducing cattle abortion when, for example, a bull had got into a field of underaged and undersized heifers. There were several bottles still on the shelf when another load arrived. Most were still there when a third load arrived. Then I found out that not only had I over ordered but a new cheaper version was being produced by another drug company. Lesson learnt: find out exactly what we use of each drug each month and buy it competitively. By this time, I was beginning to use a primitive BBC computer for my stock control and ordering and rather than ask the drug reps what we used I told them and often got a better discount. The rep who had over-egged my order got a bit of a tough time from me next time he came in, but he taught me an important lesson I never forgot.

As well as the usual cat parvovirus vaccine and dog distemper, hepatitis and lepto injection, was now added canine parvovirus. We also did the odd rabies vaccination for dogs and cats being exported but these vaccines were strictly controlled until the Pet Passport Scheme came about in 2004. Some horses were vaccinated against tetanus, but many were not, so we used a lot of antiserum on cut or injured horses. Equine flu vaccines were also available but still not widely used.

There was also a rabbit myxomatosis vaccine privately manufactured which we used, and it seemed to protect pet rabbits very well when it was used. Cattle were also vaccinated against brucellosis, using the so-called S19 vaccine, which was good at preventing the disease in cattle, but accidental self-injection caused the disease in people. So, preventing preventable disease became my motto for the next decade. My first plan was to increase uptake, as only 50% of the dogs that regularly came to the practice were vaccinated, and fewer than 35% of cats. As far as pet rabbits were concerned, we put more to sleep with "myxy" because they were not vaccinated during an outbreak than we ever vaccinated.

During the 1980s, cat flu vaccination became available and we saw more cases of cat flu than we saw with "panleuc" (panleucopaenia); although the latter was fatal, the former was often life-changing and very debilitating. The current mentality amongst vets and clients was treat rather than prevent. They obviously did not hear Mr Steele-Bodger's talk at the RVC. The vaccinations for cat flu were followed in the decade by vaccines for feline leukaemia virus and then feline chlamydia. The former is one of the few viral causes of cancer but also immunosuppressive disease in cats. Chlamydia in cats is a common cause of single or bilateral eye inflammation (conjunctivitis).

What a long hard struggle I had getting clients as well as my partners and junior vets in the practice, as the practice had grown to ten vets at its peak of farm work, to accept my preventive approach. I attacked the problem in many ways. Firstly, in the case of diseases such as feline leukaemia (FeLV), the disease itself did the trick.

As well as our branches in Marden and Headcorn, we opened in Staplehurst and Tenterden. Staplehurst was a commuter area with a large pet cat population. There seemed to be a cluster of cases of FeLV and as the number of fatal cases that were FeLV positive increased, it was obvious that we should include this vaccine with our routine cat vaccination regime in that village and if there, why not the rest of the practice? The other way I got more vaccine components on the agenda was by buying enough doses of FeLV and panleucopaenia that the chlamydia doses were given free by the drug company. Similarly, with dog vaccines I see kennel cough, a complex set of infections including parainfluenza virus (PI) and Bordetella, a close relative of whooping cough, as another disease worthy of protecting dogs against.

The final way to improve vaccine uptake and maintain regular boosters was to send clients a discount voucher with the reminders – a scheme Larry and Eric found distasteful until they saw the increased uptake and realised marketing in a veterinary practice was not a dirty word but actually improved the level of protection against preventable disease. An example of what Eric thought about marketing is shown by his comment when I said Cranbrook needed a new sign outside as the existing one had fallen over several months before, he remarked, "Everyone knows where we are," as if nobody ever moved into the practice area.

To bring the discussion right up to date, there was even a vaccine for a dog coronavirus which caused a severe haemorrhagic gastroenteritis especially if concurrent with parvovirus. We vaccinated all the puppies in the practice for the two years it was available, as it was the same price as other dog vaccines so why not use it? There must still be a group of nine- to ten-year-old dogs in the area immune to coronavirus thanks to this vaccine.

The latest vaccine update is that there are now lepto vaccines that protect against more strains, so my argument is why not use them? I certainly do not subscribe to the idea that the immune system cannot cope with more than one antigen. Nature does not work like that. One of the original vaccines I used in practice was the seven clostridial strains used to protect sheep against these diseases and then of course pasteurella pneumonia was added, making it an effective eight component vaccine for sheep – how on earth will their immune system cope?

The saying "fit as a butcher's dog" was first recorded in Victorian times and refers to butchers' dogs obviously being fed a high-quality high meat diet, particularly unusual in both the human and certainly canine population at the time. The term also suggests they may be overweight, but Butcher Bill in Marden had GSD dogs and they were all fit and not an ounce overweight, although in my opinion on a too high protein diet. They only ever had one dog at a time but over the time I have known the family the resident GSD was always called Ben and all three lived long and happy lives.

It was Ben One that had the most memorable health issue. He had a bad cut on his back leg from climbing over corrugated iron sheeting in the backyard of the butchers. This needed a full GA and about twenty stitches. All was healing well until Ben decided to chew his stitches out early so after three days needed re-stitching under local. Three of the stitches were again chewed out within 24 hours and we were forced to resort to a new idea. Buster cones are now widely used and widely recognised as a collar fitting device to prevent such wound chewing but in Ben One's time twenty years ago they were not manufactured. The idea was, however, recorded so we successfully cut the bottom out of a lightweight plastic bucket, removed the handle and fitted it to his collar when re-stitching him for the third time. The wound now healed perfectly, and the stitches removed by me ten days after the last re-stitch.

The only problem was that Bill the Butcher's yard was visible from the High Street through a gate and people kept going into the butchers telling Bill that Ben had his head stuck in a bucket!

Publicans' dogs, especially before smoking in pubs was banned in 2007, were certainly not as fit as Butcher Bill's Ben I, II or III – or most butchers' dogs. The problem is that smoke is heavier than air, so cigarette smoke is even denser at dog level and in pubs they spent their lives inhaling higher levels of cigarette smoke than any of the regulars or bar staff.

Most dogs easily become expert at food scrounging and in pubs there are many packets of snacks and plenty of punters to work on. Jenny was one very unfit pub dog; she was a collie type dog my mother would have described as a Heinz 57 (57 varieties in her genetic make-up), she was overweight and had chronic bronchitis. When I first visited her pub, I walked in wearing my usual work uniform, before the hospital scrub era, of tweed jacket and trousers, carrying my black bag and stethoscope. I walked into the pub before opening time and without looking up from the glasses he was stacking the barman called "Second on the left" and stood pointing to a door by the bar. I went through the door and second left and found myself standing in the pub's gents' toilet. I went back out to the bar and said, "That's the gents."

"Yes," said the barman, looking at me a little surprised. "But I have come to see the pub dog."

"Oh sorry," he chuckled, embarrassed by not noticing the stethoscope I had in my hand; "I was expecting the service engineer to fix the condom machine. The landlady is in the saloon bar straight down the corridor." Jenny was in there wheezing and overweight with her loving owner, also a little overweight. I advised a chest x-ray and a diet alongside antibiotics and bronchodilator tablets and she lived many wheezy years, but not long enough to see the smoking ban and needed the bronchodilator permanently along with regular antibiotics. She never did come in for the x-ray, but chronic bronchitis was definitely the diagnosis.

Another memorable pub dog was Panzer, a massive German Shepherd. His owner, the landlord of the Bull at Linton rang me at Headcorn Surgery about 9.30 one morning and said Panzer had a sore ear. I offered to go straight there but he said he had to go out but would be back at 12.30 and wanted to be there, warning that Panzer was an aggressive guard dog and not particularly good with strangers, especially vets. "Forewarned was forearmed," I thought as I knocked on the back door at 12.45. Instead of the expected landlord, I heard Panzer barking and the voice of an obviously old lady: "Just a minute, I am coming."

"Is the landlord in?" I asked, but no reply. Just the crash at the door as Panzer hit it barking aggressively. To my surprise the bolts started sliding as a little lady looked around the door. I said in a raised voice, "Don't open the door!"

She not only opened the door but stood aside, giving Panzer a clear run at me. "Oh," she said, "my son's not in," realising Panzer was about to charge at me. Panzer reminded me of the elephant charging the photographer as he came at me. I could not grab the door but just lifted my black bag expecting the full force any second.

"SIT!" I shouted at the top of my voice. He did not sit but suddenly turned and walked back into the pub. I was so surprised at his response I followed him into the saloon bar and called "Panzer come here" and to my surprise he did. "Sit," I shouted again and unbelievably he did. The little old lady was as surprised as I was. He had a collar on, and I asked her to get a lead. As she wandered off, I put the muzzle on him, repeating my instruction to "Sit". He grumbled but continued to sit.

I held his collar and checked his left ear which was normal; the right ear canal was sore and waxy. By the time the old lady came back with his lead I was massaging ear cleaner into his sore right ear, which he tolerated, and then put in some medicated drops and injected him with anti-inflammatory. I slipped off the muzzle and drove back to Cranbrook. Ten minutes later an astonished Bull landlord was on the phone. "How did you manage that?" he asked. "My mother tells me you managed Panzer quite well. How on earth did you do that?"

"He was a good obedient boy," I said; "you have trained him well." I gave further advice about treatment for his ears, but Panzer was overall certainly as fit as a butcher's dog and very obedient, I am pleased to say.

That morning I really thought I was going to add to my list of animal-related hospital visits, but all was well. Not so when dealing with a Border collie with a fractured pelvis early in my time at the Maidstone practice. The three-year-old collie was heavily sedated, but a sedative is not a general anaesthetic and I was asked by colleagues to help lift her onto the x-ray table. Perhaps the sedative dose was too low, or she just fought her way through it. The vet whose case it was lifted her back end and I took the front end. She just briefly opened her eyes, sat up and bit me through the lip. I went straight round to Maidstone Hospital and had three stitches under my lower lip.

I again needed twelve stitches in my right hand after visiting a so-called off-colour Cocker spaniel in Marden. The dog was hiding under a table and nobody in the family hinted he might bite. I offered my hand in a friendly way and the dog flew out from under the table and grabbed my right hand, ripping the skin from the base of my thumb to the bottom of the palm of my hand. "I should have told you he bites," said the owner, as I wrapped my hand in a bandage from my black bag. I then muzzled and treated the dog before heading to casualty.

The third visit came from a cattle kick. I was castrating bullocks in a cattle race at Nick's farm in Sutton Valence, approaching each bullock from behind, injecting local and then neutering them. The one that kicked me over the left eye, causing me to need five stitches over my eyebrow, had not even had its local injection when it back kicked me in the face. I felt obliged to complete the procedures on all the stock before heading to casualty as Nick and Chris, or was it Simon, were not very sympathetic.

The common theme to all three injuries was when reporting to reception at the hospital one of the questions was, "What's the problem?" Answer: "Dog bite" or "Cattle kick", and one of the next questions was "Occupation?" I guarantee that no matter what the animal-related injury, the answer "Vet" always got a vaguely unsympathetic laugh from the receptionist. Luckily, I suppose three minor stitch-ups after a long professional career in mixed practice is reasonable and at least I can see the funny side of these stories.

During my career I was sent hundreds of Christmas cards and presents from grateful clients and lots of thank-you cards and letters the rest of the time. Sadly, most of the latter were from clients thanking me after the sad passing of their pet with my help, but I did get an e-mail from a cat apologising for scratching me; however, Bembo's was the best card.

Bembo was a Springer spaniel who against the owner's wishes and mine had his tail docked at birth, been castrated by me, had a splenectomy for a benign tumour of the spleen, had a toe amputated because of a chronic nail bed infection leading to deep bone infection, and removal of benign skin tumours on multiple occasions.

The card read:

Dear Uncle John,

Are you making another dog from all the bits you keep taking from me?

Bembo

The Frankenstein's dog story could have continued as finally Bembo had a bone cancer. The aggressive treatment for this involves leg amputation and a vicious chemotherapy regime which can prolong comfortable life expectancy from just weeks to up to a year. Both his owners and I were against this and opted to let nature take its course as he was nearly ten. Surprisingly, Bembo did so well that six months after diagnosis and palliative treatment only, I asked the laboratory to check his pathology result and an orthopaedic specialist to check his x-rays. Both confirmed the diagnosis of sinister osteosarcoma but Bembo remained symptom- and pain-free for another year after this and he was close to twelve years of age.

He was one of two bone cancer patients who had a happier outcome than all the other cases I had seen where the non-amputation option meant just weeks or even just days of uncomfortable life. The end when it came was peaceful and he was a complete character even if in his and his owner's words he was not a complete dog.

One of the more memorable letters the author received during his career

19

THE HAIL CAESAR SECTION

One of the measures of success in the preservation and prolongation of life for farm and pet animals must be a reduction of the perinatal death rate of both mother and offspring.

The biggest problem with all obstetric cases is that things go wrong so quickly, and issues are not noticed or ignored and the key to a successful outcome is an early professional assessment. It is no coincidence that, for examples, the farmers who think they do not need a vet's help are the ones who end up with the least satisfactory results after they eventually call. Because the longer the problem is left, either noticed or unnoticed, the poorer the survival chances of the neonate and then eventually the mother.

During my time at Cranbrook, I could not count the number of out-of-hours calls where the duty nurse rang and informed me of a visit for calving, lambing or whelping. There were also occasional kittenings, foalings and farrowings. Some of these events occurred in normal office hours but not very often.

Here are a few memorable examples. I was called to a Doberman breeder in Hawkhurst, her four-year-old bitch was straining, and I was asked to ring her. On interrogation the dog had been off food and nestbuilding but not been straining until the last twenty minutes. The whole process sounded normal and it was the due date. It would have been easy to tell the owner to give the bitch more time, but I felt my skills might be needed. I was at the house on the green by the village hospital within thirty minutes. On my arrival, still no puppies had appeared. During my examination, the bitch's temperature was slightly low, which is often the case; on internal examination a puppy's head was felt but right at the tip of my finger. Had the bitch strained forcefully I would have just given her more time but when feeling the upper level of her birth canal the reflex strain was weak and a simple feel of the very friendly bitch's abdomen suggested more than four puppies, probably as many as six or seven. I therefore gave her an IM dose of oxytocin.

When I first qualified, only less concentrated pituitary extract was available, but the oxytocin was much more potent. Within ten minutes of the injection the first puppy was born. I checked him for any deformities such as cleft palate and passed him over to his mother's care. Within minutes a backward presented puppy was born, and the bitch cleaned herself and her two puppies frequently. An internal check proved another was on the way and twenty minutes later was born head first. About 60% of puppies are born head first, the remaining 40% tail first. Half an hour before the next puppy, a further examination showed her contractions were weakening again. This was a classic case of uterine (womb) inertia where birth contractions are weaker and in some extreme cases non-existent.

I repeated the oxytocin injection and waited another twenty minutes when on internal I could feel another puppy in the canal. My digital exploration and the puppy's presence encouraged straining and v-sign fingers around the puppy's head gave me the leverage to pull it down and out. I have never used forceps to deliver puppies or kittens. Another live normal puppy. Another swiftly followed, then within ten minutes another. The process continued and within an hour there were six live puppies born and more to come. I discussed the advantages and disadvantages of doing a caesarean if needed. The advantage may be an increased chance of more live puppies but the disadvantages are of surgical and anaesthetic risks to the mother and the new-born and unborn.

We decided to continue and within the next hour one live and one dead puppy were born. The bitch was content feeding her seven puppies and it had been a long night. I was sure a caesarean section would not have saved the dead puppy as it also seemed smaller than its littermates. A long night and a successful one, we all felt. I gave the happy mother a course of antibiotic to prevent post-whelping womb or mammary infection and one last shot of oxytocin to close her womb down and expel any remaining afterbirth as no more puppies could be felt. I was wrong about there being seven puppies instead of eight, but I was right about not rushing into a caesarean.

Unresponsive uterine inertia was not the only reason for this common procedure, there were other causes for this life saving operation.

A caesarean was certainly needed when years later one of our vets wanted to just keep giving oxytocin to a whelping Cavalier King Charles spaniel. The dog was four years old and called Molly. He could feel a puppy in the canal and gave oxytocin but when that did not produce a puppy was willing to keep the dog hospitalised overnight and re-assess it in the morning. This may have been all right if after a long discussion with the owner they should jointly decide to postpone further treatment and go to any length to avoid a caesarean, but that had not happened. The duty nurse was so concerned I was called in at midnight and the duty vet was happy to get my opinion.

I examined the bitch: a puppy was engaged in the canal and I was sure there were more than one. I could have carried out an ultrasound, but I was in no doubt a caesarean was necessary, so I rang Helen, Molly's owner, and got permission. A general anaesthetic (GA) using drugs kindest to the puppies was chosen, then a midline abdominal incision and a single uterine cut allowed two live puppies to be born by squeezing them through the same wound toothpaste-style; they were behind a dead monster puppy with a massive, deformed head that was blocking their normal exit. That was also removed through the existing womb incision. Without a caesarean that night the two puppies would probably have been dead by morning and even Molly's life and certainly breeding potential risked if left longer than 48 hours. The womb was then stitched, followed by the abdomen, as the live puppies were revived and checked for congenital defects.

These two cases clearly show the options available with modern veterinary obstetrics for dogs and similar options are available for cats kittening – but what about cattle. I have discussed several calving cases but often the calf cannot be born, leaving just two options. Embryotomy, the cutting up of a dead calf inside the cow, or caesarean. Firstly, let us talk about the former. I was called up the road to my friend Graham when I lived next door to his farm in Headcorn. The cow calving had a head back and unlike Morri's cow the calf was dead. I got a head rope around the head but even with an epidural could not straighten the head or get the legs back to get a normal dive position. The answer was to pass an embryotomy wire around the dead calf's neck, pass the two ends through a protective tube called an embryotomy tube, then decapitate the calf inside the cow without damaging the cow. The calf's head was then pulled out of the cow and I could then rope and pull the two front legs and the decapitated body out of the cow. The benefits to the cow were this was less traumatic than a caesarean and this proved to be the case as the cow made a good recovery and continued to have a calf a year for several years.

As far as the many cow caesars in my career are concerned, two again stand out. The first one was at a dairy farm in Hollingbourne owned by the Leggat family. Larry was already on the farm doing a caesarean on one cow when they called again with another calving. Both cows had been inseminated by the same bull. Larry was stitching up the womb of his cow when I got there and told me his calf had been just too big for the cow's pelvis but was now born by caesar alive and well.

It did not take many minutes of trying to calve mine before I felt this calf was also too big for normal birth. I clipped the cow's left flank, injected local around the spinal nerves as they emerged in the lumbar spinal region, and cut in through the skin and muscle layers. I pushed the rumen aside and exposed the uterus. All with the cow standing. I cut into the uterus and pulled out another massive live calf to grow up with Larry's. The wounds were sutured and both cows made good recoveries with routine post-operative care and regular visits from either Larry or me. A call was also made to the Artificial Insemination Centre reporting the bull for siring such large calves.

The other memorable cattle caesar was one I did for Farmer Reynolds in Hawkhurst. I was called because they could not make head nor tail of a calving. On examination I could feel a solid V-shaped calf and intestines. First, I considered a tear of the uterus allowing the cow's guts in, or a deformed calf with a massive umbilical hernia. Then I remembered Professor Arthur talking about a bovine deformity called Schistosoma reflexes. The calves cannot be born due to a solid spine and an inside-out abdomen. The cow can be saved by a caesarean so that is what I did.

20

BROKEN HEARTS

In 1980 my world fell apart and I was devastated. It was in March: just as the darkness of winter lifted my own darkness descended as my wife left me and took my almost two-year-old son Ross with her. As the evenings got lighter, I sat amongst the daffodils, by the pond I had just fenced off to protect my son, contemplating how you can try and see the future and protect your loved ones from harm but some things you just do not see coming.

I felt so low and determined not to harm myself so refused to have any barbiturates or the gun in my car overnight in case the deep dark pit of despair overwhelmed me. I knew the suicide rate amongst vets was high and had recently overtaken farmers. One of the complex reasons was easy access to the means.

Several years later I was skiing on a vet conference and seven of us were sat around a bar and the conversation got to this devastating statistic. As one of my colleagues at Tom's had killed himself, I then pulled the metaphorical hand-grenade pin and threw it in. "Have any of you guys or girls contemplated suicide?"

One by one they replied "No" until I got to John, my colleague from Dorking, who said, "Yes, I am from a small mining town in Scotland and I am gay!" He then opened up in detail how he knew his sexuality but somehow it never worked out and he had considered the permanent solution to a temporary problem.

It was quite an experience being there when someone "comes out" and we all reassured John that he would find happiness in the end. I also said to him, "John, if you ever feel really down ring me any time day or night." He assured me he would. Years later John was found dead in a Thai hotel where he was working for a veterinary charity and the Thai coroner said it was liver failure. I certainly hope so, but John had always seemed fit to me and was when I last saw him before he went cycling around the Far East.

To fight the darkness surrounding me, I went to see my parents on my day off that March. They were living in a bungalow at Kingswood just opposite the Battle of Britain pub at the time My father was inevitably like me always working so quickly left my mother and me over a cup of tea. My mother, in her usual philosophical way, looked at me over her teacup and asked, "How old are you now?" Knowing full well how old I was. "I'm thirty," I told her. "I am 68 and would just love to be thirty again," she said. It was very much: you have a lovely son, get on and enjoy your life and do not regret anything. As the song goes, "Mama said you can't hurry love!" I looked out of the window and over to the same Battle of Britain pub we vet students had scurried by pushing the papier-mâché animals all those years before and knew I did not want to re-live or change anything.

Mickey Finn (yes, the owners' surname is Finn) was an 11-month-old neutered black and white cat when he was presented at Headcorn surgery one morning as a routine appointment. He was breathing badly, and examination showed several scuffed nails suggesting he had been hit by a car. The sound from his chest was very dull when it was tapped with a pair of fingers. No heart sounds could be heard through a stethoscope and his tummy seemed very empty. His mouth was open as he breathed, and he was most distressed if tilted forwards. All classic signs of a ruptured diaphragm after an RTA (road traffic accident). He would need surgery to repair the injury as soon as possible.

Back in the theatre at Cranbrook after the diagnosis was confirmed on an x-ray, he was given oxygen for twenty minutes by holding a mask near his face but not panicking him. Keeping him upright seemed to help his breathing. His hair was clipped for a midline abdominal incision and the skin partially scrubbed. Then the moment of truth: he was given a sedative followed by an injectable anaesthetic. He was quickly intubated with an ET so the nurse could pump his lungs by pressing on the external bag. After a final scrub of both of us, I made a long midline abdominal incision. I could see into his chest cavity and in there were loads of his intestines and his liver. No wonder I could not hear his heart with the stethoscope earlier. I quickly but gently pulled his intestines, then his liver, back into his abdomen. His collapsed lungs were now in sight in front of his heart, both visible through a large tear in his diaphragm, the muscle between his chest and abdominal cavities.

The nurse's role was vital. Inflate, I said, and she gently puffed air into Mickey's collapsed lungs, and they inflated in front of my eyes; gently we re-expanded his lungs so they filled his chest cavity. Between each positive pressure breath in, the lungs would partially collapse with a negative pressure breath out by releasing the squeeze on the anaesthetic bag. I gathered together the tattered edges of the diaphragm and could only stitch when he was breathing out for fear of penetrating the tiny needle with its attached suture material into his expanded lungs. Starting deepest towards his back, a stitch was inserted and the deepest torn edge of the diaphragm re-aligned. Between breaths and with the nurse breathing him out each time, a stitch went in the muscle and the rupture was repaired. Once it was clear the repair was down to the last stitch, it was not tied until a big inflation puff to expel as much air from the chest cavity before that last stitch was pulled together and tied. The abdominal wound was then quickly repaired. Once his chest was closed, he wanted to breathe for himself, but the nurse assisted. A 20ml syringe and catheter with a three-way tap was used to make sure no air was left in his chest. Mickey made a great recovery and was discharged home two days later, leaving him just eight lives of his original nine!

One evening I was on duty and got a couple of calls. My friend Nick was lodging with me at the time and offered to help. I told him to bring his wellies. The first was a trip to Cranbrook to see a cat in an RTA. The nails were scuffed but the cat was lying uncomfortably and walked with a very rolling action. A full physical examination was normal until I placed my two thumbs on each side of its waist. There was a characteristic click of crepitus, as felt in Dave's clavicle when he broke it playing football at college all those years before. "He has broken his pelvis," I said. An x-ray confirmed a minor fracture of the pelvis which would heal with 4-6 weeks rest, providing there were no complications.

The next call was to a Friesian cow at Hole Park Farm, Rolvenden, with milk fever, the classic lack of calcium after calving. I examined her with Nick holding the calcium bottle IV drip high as I guided the needle into the jugular vein. It was then Nick asked, "Have you checked her pelvis?" The cow was certainly lying in a remarkably similar position to the cat and I saw exactly what Nick meant. I laughed and replied, "Yes, an orthopaedic check is a major part of a 'down cow' examination."

Nick was most impressed when at the end of the drip ten minutes later the cow stood up.

I had a great single life for the next six years. I was a good part-time father and had lots of girlfriends, some serious and some not so serious. Then in 1986, boom, I met Sandra. She worked for the practice insurance brokers and for Ian and Anne in their pub most evenings and we chatted the night of Ian and Anne's ten years in The Bell celebration which was a Wednesday night. The following Saturday night my girlfriend and I went to a different pub, the Three Chimneys, for a meal and what a surprise to see Sandra working a night there as well. The girlfriend I was with remarked, "She seems a nice girl," – but was more than a little put out when I agreed.

I had managed to get tickets to an INXS concert at Hammersmith and to Wimbledon tennis so rang my brokers and invited Sandra. I was incredibly pleased when she accepted, and we were virtually inseparable with her even coming on visits with me whilst on duty. One of these was to a farrowing. I clearly remember it was at a pig farm in Hawkenbury during June 1986. It is all very well finding a young lady willing to come to a concert and go to Wimbledon, but to a pig farm is a real litmus test of any relationship. A farrowing is like a mixture of a lambing and a whelping. The sow had not managed to produce any piglets but was straining and her cervix was open; on internal examination I managed to grab hold of a piglet and pull it out, this was followed by two or three others all within arm's reach. The pregnant uterus of a sow consists of two horns, the left and the right. I emptied both horns as far as I could reach lying down behind the sow, but the horns then bent downwards with 180 degree turn and although from the weight I knew there were piglets, I could not reach them. I injected oxytocin and waited ten minutes when the sow started straining again and another five piglets were reachable. On a final internal examination, no more piglets could be felt but I warned there might be more out of reach, but the uterus felt less heavy and I thought she had finished. I warned the farmer that I thought there could easily be another hidden. I gave the sow one last injection of oxytocin and some antibiotic, but she had finished and made a great recovery, rearing all nine piglets. Not a big litter but a healthy one and a great test of any courtship.

In late September, my mother came unannounced to my Headcorn surgery with two of her dogs for "vaccination". I took one look at the vaccination certificates and thought they were in date. "Well, I wanted a word. Have you got a minute?" she asked. I walked her to the car. My dad was of course working. Off she went with a very strange comment, "When are you going to marry Sandra?" When I embarrassingly replied about "plenty of time", she told me, "There is not plenty of time. Tony must come all the way from Australia, and I am not getting any younger!"

The following Saturday I got a call from my father. He was too choked to speak, passing me to an ambulance driver who said, "Your mother has had a heart attack; I am afraid she is dead!"

I got engaged to Sandra the following Christmas and married her in the following June, not because my mother suggested it but because I wanted to and "There is not plenty of time!" Between the engagement and the wedding, it was lambing time again and Sandra came whenever she could join me on visits. One of which was to Cranbrook where sometimes farmers would drop off lambings into our stables and we would deal with them when back from other calls.

One night there was a ewe with a prolapse. Cows and ewes get two sorts of prolapse: vaginal before birth and uterine after. The former group are simply replaced and sometimes need suturing in place. The sutures need removing during the birthing process. The latter, uterine prolapses, are much more difficult to deal with but easier in the ewe as they can be upturned, and gravity helps prevent straining as the organ is replaced. Nonetheless, it is a spectacular and bloody process even in the ewe and then the vulva is sutured as with vaginal prolapses. Sandra watched unphased as the life of the mother of a pair of twin lambs was saved by this dramatic technique.

The wedding was a lovely sunny day in June 1987 and my best man was Graham, the farmer neighbour whose uncle had helped me with the finances in South Africa and a lifelong friend. He had now sold his Headcorn farm and lived in a flat overlooking Tenterden where Sandra also lived. In his best man speech, he described how about a year before I had looked out of his window and remarked, "The lady of my dreams is out there somewhere."

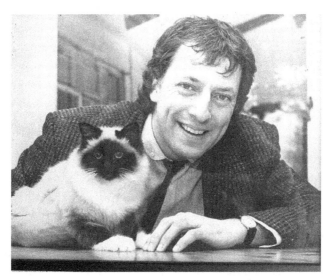

The author with feline companion Alf in 1989

"Little did we know Sandra lived over the road from my flat," he said. My father was at the wedding and thoroughly enjoyed the event. My Aunt Joan was also there. It was she who had rung me when my mother died the previous year saying that at least she did not suffer, going so suddenly. She had assured me that was far better than slowly and drawn out which was exactly what happened to her in October 1987 with uterine cancer – and then my father. He had a complicated cancer and was in hospital for several weeks, slowly deteriorating after several surgeries and false dawns. During his stay in hospital, I went to see him every day and although he and I were never as close as I was to my mother, I did love him, and we did understand each other's quite different views on life.

On one of the occasions I went to visit him he was fast asleep, so I left him a note. My handwriting is bad, so in it I said if he could not read it to get it taken to the pharmacy and see if they gave him anything interesting. One of the nurses and he finally managed to translate what I had said, and it certainly caused a laugh amongst the nurses. Sadly, they did have to use a lot of morphine on him and on one visit he told me it was "The best cruise he had ever been on," pointing at the nurse behind the console at the end of the ward saying, "What a great captain they have running the ship!" In a way he was correct. Sadly, he died on 17th May 1989 but not before my two brothers had come to say goodbye, Tony flying in from Australia.

On 3rd October 1991, our first baby was due – a half sibling to Ross. We made the mistake of buying an Indian takeout and watching a video. The film was "Pacific Heights" starring Melanie Griffiths and Michael Keaton. It was a memorable film in which Melanie Griffiths and Mathew Modine, as a young couple, take in a lodger to help finance their beautiful house. The lodger is Michael Keaton, the tenant from Hell. It was a memorable film as Sandra went into labour half-way through it. We had all the scan pictures and I even had a video of our baby taken with our ultrasound machine from the practice but wanted to keep our baby's sex a surprise, so I had not looked at some details of the pictures and film.

Sandra rang the hospital and they said that as the labour pains were not too frequent to leave it an hour and then get into Maidstone Hospital Maternity Unit. We watched the rest of the film and as Sandra's bag was already packed, we just loaded the car and set off. It was a long night. I had prepared a tape cassette of all Sandra's favourite music and this was soon being played by the midwife as Sandra went into full labour. We regretted the curry as she was extremely sick in the night. "Perhaps a lighter supper would have been better," said the midwife, as she took away the bucket. The labour was very painful even for me as Sandra squeezed my hand so tight. Pain relief for her included gas and air and a failed epidural, and for me running my squashed hand under cold water! By mid-day on Friday 4th we were told there was a mal-presentation and instead of baby facing her mother she was facing backwards and as engaged in the canal was too late to move around.

The consultant was called, and he popped his head around the door about 2pm, took one look from where he stood, and said, "You are a big, tall girl, you will manage." This left the midwife huffing, as well as my wife who in fact has a very skinny waist. Another failed epidural and an hour later the consultant was off duty and the midwife called the duty surgeon who quite rightly decided to do a caesarean. The midwife promised I could attend theatre but then the anaesthetist was reluctant so bravely Sandra said, "I am not signing a consent form unless my husband can be there." Eventually, when the midwife again promised I could attend, Sandra signed the consent form, unbelievably commenting on the house surgeon's very neat fountain pen saying, "Nice pen!"

We went to the operating theatre after prepping Sandra for the c. section and I had to wait in the changing room. Within ten minutes I was called into theatre as Sandra's womb was being stitched in front of me whilst Sandra was under full general anaesthetic as the epidurals had not worked – and the midwife was holding my daughter. I said, "How did you get me in?" She replied, "I called for a paediatrician." When one did not arrive she announced to the surgical and anaesthetic team, "I will get a vet instead." I helped bathe, clean and weigh my daughter before Sandra was awake. I even have a photo of me in scrubs with her in before her mother woke up. When she was awake and cuddling her baby, Sandra's parents and sister arrived. As we left the hospital, Bruce, my father-in-law, asked if anyone fancied a curry. I declined, and we opted for a pizza.

Jake's birth was equally exciting. He was due on 1st April but was heading to be over two weeks late. The second week was the vet conference in Birmingham and very handily I had two tickets for the cup semi-final just down the road at Villa Park between Manchester United and Crystal Palace. I had planned to go with Ross, but Jake had other plans. He was due to be induced on the Monday, but my pager went off on the Friday so I rushed out of lectures to find a call box. The call was just a routine call from the practice, but I felt it might be a bit of a rush to get back from Birmingham so ended up watching the team lose on TV on the Sunday, but the induction went ahead on the Monday. Interestingly, the drug used for induction included prostaglandin, the drug that was unheard of when I was at college, and the same oxytocin drug we used in veterinary obstetrics. Jake was born after a long, hard but normal labour and has been a lifelong Crystal Palace supporter. Our daughter Rhianna was born on 4th October 1991 and Jake followed on 10th April 1995. That too has a symmetry: 4/10 and 10/4. All made more poignant by the fact they were both born in the hospital where my father had died.

During this period, dog and cat work took more and more of my time and the farm and equine side less. Out of hours I still did my share. Radio-pagers meant I could be on duty and not need to be by a phone. I had a mental map of all the coinbox phones in the area and could be in touch with the nurses at Cranbrook within minutes of the bleeper firing off. This meant more freedom on first call or second call and even allowed me to play tennis more. The bleepers then had short messages and by the late 1990s mobile phones were available, negating the need for using phone boxes.

Livestock farming was in decline in the area and our new assistant

Duncan was very keen on doing the limited work that was available, leaving me free to pursue the dog and cat work. He became a partner in 1998 and Doug retired in 1999. As well as my interest in general surgery I became extremely interested in dental surgery. Dental disease in dogs and cats is quite common and gum disease a real welfare and ongoing issue. I became an active member of the British Veterinary Dental Association and learnt so much on courses on how to prevent gum disease in dogs and cats as well as sophisticated tooth fracture repair using light-cured materials, correct extraction techniques and even root canals and pulp treatments. This was a logical extension of my belief in preventive medicine. Why just extract bad teeth from dogs and cats? Better to prevent tooth problems by feeding proper preventive diets and regular dental prophylaxis.

In 1986 my interest in cardiology also continued and again I attended many lectures and courses. At one of the big veterinary conferences, an American veterinary cardiologist was lecturing on the use of ECGs in dogs. I had done a bit of work using one at college on my cattle pericarditis case, so I was stimulated enough to try and understand the electrical waves over the heart a little better. After the lecture I bought his standard textbook and started doing ECGs on my cardiac patients once I persuaded the other partners to let me purchase a machine. It soon paid for itself and the standard of cardiac care in the practice increased with much earlier investigation of our cardiac cases and more tailored treatments, leading to better survival rates. A big increase in Mr Steele-Bodger's middle triage group.

In the summer of 1988, I fitted my first pacemaker into a dog. Poppy was a little terrier that kept collapsing because she had a usual heart rate of under 40 beats per minute. This was adequate when resting but the moment she exercised that was too slow and the little dog passed out. I managed to obtain a second-hand pacemaker from Maidstone Hospital thanks to the consultant cardiologist, as they were often removed from her patients for various reasons. I just had to get an estimate of the lead cost from the company as a new intravenous pacing lead would be needed. The owners managed to find the cost for this, and the operation was booked.

Usually, to fit the cable a fluoroscope was needed to check the position of the pacer lead within the right ventricle, which was passed down the jugular vein into the heart, but I devised an ECG system. The ECG lead was attached to the pacer lead and a characteristic intraventricular ECG obtained. The position of the lead was confirmed by a series of x-rays. Several plates showed the lead in the right top chamber, called the right atrium, and several too far through out into the pulmonary arteries but finally in the right ventricular wall. The pacemaker unit was connected at a fixed rate of 100 beats per minute. It was buried under the skin in front of her right shoulder and Poppy lived a long and happy life. Her owners always attended my ECG courses all over the country where her spectacular paced heartbeat produced some wonderful ECG traces from the delegates' practical sessions.

After mastering the ECG machine, I was attending another cardiology course in Antwerp, Belgium, given by another American cardiologist and chatted to him during a coffee break as to how I could persuade the partners to go to the next level and afford a cardiac ultrasound machine, which would literally let us see into diseased cats' and dogs' hearts. The expense was phenomenal but instead of the usual accountant's view of costing equipment with how quickly a piece of equipment paid for itself, his view was that if it improved the practice's clinical standard and kept me interested in doing a professional job at a high standard, it was worthwhile. I agreed but sold it to my partners on the accountant's view of cost repaid over how many years.

All three views were correct and we purchased an ultrasound machine in 1991: this raised the clinical standard of cardiac diagnosis, it put me on a whole new learning curve and paid for itself very quickly. The use for other clinical work such as pregnancy and abdominal work was a bonus. Sandra was pregnant with Rhi at this time and during all the trials as to which ultrasound machine we should buy I got some great video footage at a time most mums-to-be just got a still picture.

I then took and passed further qualification in cardiology and started seeing referrals of cardiac cases from other practices, including faxed ECGs from all over the country and from my ex-partner, Mel, who was now working in Saudi Arabia. The idea that I should offer the fax referral service to other practices came whist chatting to my friend Douglas who was the owner of several veterinary publications. He encouraged me to write articles promoting this service. At the time many vet cardiologists were offering trans-telephonic ECGs using modified telephone systems, but none were getting actual ECGs faxed from practices. My system encouraged the practices to take their own ECGs and only send the abnormal ones, once they could recognise normal. In my opinion a great advance in veterinary education.

That Christmas I was shopping in London and by chance I bumped into one of the drug company representatives who we did quite a lot of business with. His company manufactured antibiotics in Northern Ireland and their prices were much lower than many of the brand leaders, so I knew him well. Over a beer I told him about my ECG machine and our new referral caseload and faxed ECG referrals. He said he and his wife were launching a veterinary education course module and would I like to run an ECG one? I accepted and did not think any more about it and went off down Regent Street.

I had just managed to finish my Christmas shopping in King's Road when an old dirty car pulled up alongside me flashing their CID police badges. Did I have time to attend Chelsea Police Station and help with an investigation? I jumped in the car and joined a mixed group in the police station. There were at least three postmen from the neighbouring sorting office all in their Post Office uniform, me and another older man. I was the youngest there. The detectives who had collected me off the street asked if we would help with a "line-up". They told us their suspect had as good as confessed to a crime, but the line-up would confirm it. We all agreed and were taken to a room by the duty sergeant and lined up.

A young, extremely dangerous looking young man was brought in in handcuffs and told he could stand where he liked in the line. He chose to stand next to me and the handcuffs removed. He was about 5ft 6in and almost all of us towered over him, except the postmen on the other side of us. A Belgrave Square, Chelsea-set gent was then brought in the room and the line-up sergeant said, "On the night of 29th November your home was broken into, your wife tied to a chair and you were beaten by four men and goods to the value of £10,000 taken. Do you recognise one of those men here?"

The gent walked along the line, got to my little friend and had looked at none of us until then. He then looked him in the eye, his gaze was returned coldly and, in my opinion, threateningly. So coldly that the gent averted his eyes. Without checking the last couple in the line-up, he turned on his heels saying, "I don't recognise anyone here."

The gent was led out; the handcuffs were replaced and the suspect led out. The CID officers who were not allowed to be present during the line-up were furious. There was no doubt the gent had been visually threatened, and it was not worth upsetting this gang of thugs – he and his wife had been through enough. It is no wonder line-ups are now done so the suspect cannot see the identifier and allow such obvious intimidation. An open and shut case had just been blown wide open.

The next year I ran several ECG courses with machines loaned by the company I had bought both our ECG and ultrasound machine from. The third of these was at Maidstone; there were several dogs and I usually took my very placid Birman Alf to these courses. That morning he was out hunting and instead I took my other Birman, cat Mo, who was slightly feistier. Nonetheless, all the groups got great normal ECGs from the dogs and abnormal ones from Mo. When the first group presented her ECG, I thought they had connected the leads incorrectly, but each group got the same results. Her ECG was abnormal. Later that week echocardiography (cardiac ultrasound) proved she had a thickened heart (hypertrophic cardiomyopathy – HCM). She was completely symptom-free and I had the usual dilemma as to any benefit from treatment if no symptoms, which is controversial.

Given her temperament, we decided against treatment but our lovely five-year-old had a heart attack and died within the year. After teaching this course, I got to teach both dentistry and cardiology throughout the country and was even invited to Australia to launch a heartworm preventive and talk about practice management. Perhaps my school careers officer was correct: I should have been a teacher as when I had found things difficult, I could understand a student's difficulty. Then provide short easy steps to an in-depth understanding of complicated things such as veterinary dentistry, veterinary cardiology and especially ECGs.

Alf was also another example of how modern therapy can prolong life. When Alf was due his booster, I gave him a full check-up and noticed his breathing rate was higher than normal and chest percussion and compression suggested his thoracic cavity was consolidated. Radiography the next day suggested an intra-thoracic lymphoma. Chest needle sampling proved he had chest lymphoma. I had recently been on a chemotherapy further education course, so was able to give Alf leading-edge chemotherapy which would have been unheard of a few years before. Alf was seven years old when he started on chemotherapy. He quickly went into remission and within six weeks he no longer needed weekly IV injections and went on a tablet-only regime.

Chemotherapy in dogs and cats in most cases is very unlike human chemo in that it is overall non-aggressive. Quality of life is paramount, as opposed to longevity. So, the aim is to be side-effect free with no hair loss, vomiting or other downsides. A year in the life of a dog or cat is an exceptionally long time and a large percentage of the pet's normal lifespan; therefore, overall a gentle low-dosed regime free of side-effects is preferred to an "all guns blazing", life-at-any-cost approach. Alf responded well for three years, then his chest lymphoma became resistant to therapy and I referred him to a veterinary oncologist in Cambridge. Dr Jane Dobson saw Alf and it was decided to give up on chemotherapy and use radiotherapy. He went weekly to the Cambridge vet school for six weeks, then again went into complete remission. Alf was finally euthanased with non-lymphoma renal failure at thirteen years of age.

Dead on arrival (DOA) is a sad term for when a patient fails to arrive alive at medical help. Although I saw it many times – always a sad event – among my most memorable two occasions were when I drove an hour out of Rotherham when I was locuming there, around the motorways to the other side of Sheffield to confirm a little Jack Russell tragically hit by a car was indeed dead. The owners were so obviously distressed they needed my professional opinion. As the parents of young kids, I suspect they wanted me to confirm to them all that the little dog was deceased and had not suffered. I arrived at their house, stethoscope in hand. The cadaver was still warm; it had a broken jaw and blood around its mouth and had obviously been hit in the head. No heartbeat and no breathing confirmed the animal was indeed dead.

I asked if the driver had stopped and they said, "No, just the screech of tyres after the dog had got under the front gate and the driver did not look, just drove off." I offered my condolences and offered to take her for burial or cremation, but they wanted to bury her.

Another memorable DOA was when I went to the Three Chimneys in Sissinghurst to meet Graham for a drink after he had been combine harvesting, so it must have been late August or early September. I had no sooner arrived than the phone behind the bar went for me as this was prior to pagers and mobile phones. The duty nurse told me the owners said their cat had not moved off the chair for three days and wanted it seen. To save ringing from the pub bar I took the owner's number and went to the call box outside the pub. The owners assured me the cat was breathing but had not moved for three days. I agreed to see it immediately at the Headcorn surgery which was near where they lived. I rushed back to Headcorn and opened the surgery. The 14-year-old cat was in a box and as they lifted it out it was obvious to me the cat was not only dead and in rigor mortis but had been in it long enough for the stiffness to be wearing off.

I informed them their poor cat was dead. "But it is breathing," they said. I replied, "It is not!" as this very dead, beginning to decompose, cat lay on the consulting room table. "It is breathing," they said as they lifted its head, then laid it down. There was a distinct huffing sound as the dead thorax sucked in air as a result of post-mortem change. I gently reassured the owners their cat was dead; they were still in partial denial although acceptance dawned enough to leave the cat with me.

Earlier we mentioned Mickey the cat with a ruptured diaphragm and his auscultation finding of no heart sounds: that is also exactly what I found when I examined Yogi, a 10-year-old golden retriever. He had been taken ill three days before and he saw an emergency vet at his home practice, but nothing was found wrong with him. As well as no heart sounds and fluid in his abdomen, ultrasound examination, also called echocardiography, showed his heart was surrounded by fluid as well as his abdomen. About 180ml of non-clotting blood was drained from his pericardial (membrane surrounding heart) sac; this was through a cardiac cannula placed in the fluid under local anaesthetic with Yogi fully conscious and behaving very well. The fluid in his abdomen was also drained. These pericardial effusions are spontaneous bleeds into the pericardium either due to tumours or so-called idiopathic (unknown) cause. In Yogi's case fortunately, it was the latter cause, and he made a complete recovery after just the single incident. Some idiopathic cases need several drainages and some even need the pericardial sac removed surgically and I have done this with great results apart from one Saluki Sheba who continued to need regular drainage from her chest cavity for a year but finally died from her ongoing chest effusion.

The most spectacular case was an extremely aggressive GSD which was brought in collapsed and near death by the duty vet and his owner. Echo showed the collapsing heart due to the pressure from the surrounding fluid. In his case, 150ml of non-clotting blood was drained from around his heart and as his circulation got going he stood up with the catheter still in his heart and lunged at me, blaming me for all his problems. Luckily, his owner was present and she quickly pulled him back and nobody got hurt as I grabbed the cannula from his chest. Thankfully, that was also a one-off idiopathic case. Sadly, as I say about half of these cases are sinister, most often due to blood cancers, and they have noticeably short survival times.

Unlike human cardiology, in which many heart cases are treated surgically, most veterinary heart cases are only treated medically. Humans get coronary artery disease, and many major congenital and non-congenital defects are now regularly treated surgically but, as I say, these treatments are rare, and rarely performed in our patients. However, rare does not mean non-existent. And these odd cardiac surgical cases along with some surgical respiratory cases meant I became quite slick at thoracotomies (open chest surgery). I usually approached these cases from the side most likely to give most easy access or more information.

For example, pericardectomies (removal of the pericardial sac) were usually approached from the right side between the ribs as this would give a better view of any possible tumours of the right top chamber, a favoured site for malignant haemangiosarcoma. Sometimes these would be visible on pre-operative ultrasound but not always. Sadly, if found, the owner's consent was obtained for euthanasia as it was inoperable. If a lung problem, the surgery would be performed on the relevant lung side.

One of the surgeries I frequently performed was for congenital abnormal blood vessel ligation (tying off). The most common was for PDA (patent ductus arteriosus). In the normal unborn this vessel runs from the pulmonary artery to the aorta so blood bypasses the functionless lungs. This vessel should close down around birth, so the lungs receive their full blood supply after expansion and breathing commences but, if this does not occur, blood then flows in the other direction, so the lungs are flooded with blood from the aorta.

Twist was a seven-month-old GSD cross collie referred because she was symptom free but had the machinery sounding heart murmur typical of this problem. If neglected, these cases usually do not make old bones. The treatment of choice at the time was surgery. The chest was opened on the left side with the same positive pressure technique used on Mickey with his ruptured diaphragm to keep Twist's lungs inflated. The gap between the ribs was forced as wide as possible using retractors and the lungs obstructing the view to the major vessels packed out of the way so Twist could only breathe through the right lung lobes. The patent vessel was identified running between the aorta and the pulmonary artery. The blood shunting through it could be felt with the fingertip as a machinery vibration over the pounding aorta. The vessel was gently dissected and some curved tissue forceps gently worked between the aorta and the PDA. One slip now and Twist would have bled out in seconds as the pulmonary artery and the PDA are very thin-walled blood vessels. A loop of suture material picked up and passed under the PDA allowed two ligatures to be placed each end of the PDA, making sure they did not cheese wire through the vessel. As the first of the two ties was knotted, the tremor could no longer be felt, just the normal pulse of the aorta and the pulmonary artery. The second tie was to ensure the shunt did not re-open. With the second ligature in place, it was time to reinflate the lungs fully.

There were times during the surgery when at the nurse's request the lungs were allowed a little inflation just to keep the dog's oxygenation level up as shown on the pulse oximeter. So now the rib opening needed closing as the lungs were fully re-inflated. The rib retractors had stretched the chest opening so widely that closure was not easy. The answer was to suture the two ribs together with a pair of temporary sutures to just pull the ribs together and then put the repair sutures into the incised intercostal muscles before removing the temporary sutures. Before closing the chest, the plan was to expand the lungs as much as possible and place a chest drain to allow fluid and air to be removed post-op. Twist woke up well and was kept in hospital on pain relief and the drain which was clamped off to prevent air going in and collapsing the lungs was sucked clear using a large syringe every hour initially in the first twelve hours, then every three hours. The drainage continued and Twist stayed in intensive care for three days when her experienced owner took over her care, including drainage and air suction. A week later the drain was removed, and Twist still had no sign of the machinery murmur or any murmur. Check echo showed no leakage through the surgery site. I last saw Twist seven years later and she was a happy, normal dog with no murmur and as far as I know continued to live a long and happy life.

Within a few years, some dogs were having their PDA sealed by coils passed down the aorta and released into their shunts, so I always offered this latest development at specialist referral centres. Similarly, after inserting about three pacemakers I decided it would be better for the clients to go to facilities with better surgical capabilities as these became available. After my last pacemaker insertion, a local journalist got hold of the story and the headline board outside the Cranbrook newsagents read "Vet Saves Lady's Life". This was totally misleading. The fact that Lady was the dog's name was hidden inside the article.

Perhaps my most interesting chest surgery case was a fictitious one but nonetheless based on real cases I had seen. In September 2008 I got a call from the BBC which had made no contact since I was a fifteen-year-old in one of their programmes. They were given my name by a vet with close links to the media, named John, who was in practice in Plymouth. They needed help with a script for their medical soap "Holby City". They said I would be needed to write and film the scene. The scene they wanted help with is briefly summarised as follows. The consultant chest surgeon takes his much-loved large breed dog to the hospital and leaves it in his car in the car park. During a break in his operations, he lets the dog out and it is run over by an ambulance when running in the hospital approach road. With its chest very severely injured internally, he takes it into theatre and repairs the damage and the dog makes a complete recovery.

I was asked a simple question initially: "What injury would the dog have and how would the surgeon treat this hypothetical case?" My comments were surely he would call a vet and it would be against hospital rules and medical ethics to treat the dog! After several phone conversations it was agreed that the dog would have a collapsed lung and a vet would be called. The main script writers then wrote in a non-speaking vet part in which the vet visits the roadside, shakes his head in a negative way and leaves the dog to die.

I pointed out the ethics of a real vet doing this was highly unlikely. Either the dog would be put to sleep or the vet would take the dog back to his clinic. I knew any variation of this would cast my loved profession in a very unsatisfactory light. Another compromise was reached. The vet is given a speaking part and the surgeon offers to drive the dog to the vet clinic, so the vet leaves and the surgeon then takes the dog to the basement of the hospital and drains the air from the dog's chest in a manner I described, thereby re-expanding the collapsed lungs and treating the so-called pneumothorax. In the end my defence of both medical and veterinary ethics cost me a good relationship with the BBC and I did not get to witness the filming or a mention in the credits. No wonder my phone has not rung since, apart from a local news story about dog vaccination, but I did get paid more than the three guineas my parents got for my school play.

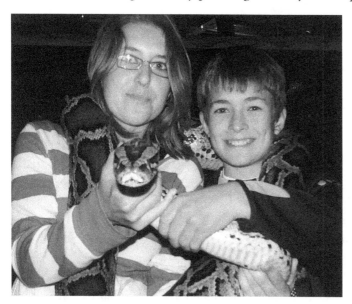

John and Sandra's children Rhianna and Jake with a friendly snake

21

SILENCE OF THE LAMBS

The year 2001 was a tough year for UK tourism and agriculture because of the foot-and-mouth disease (FMD) outbreak. As I said, by now my main work was with dogs and cats but by March the outbreak was so severe that our large animal vets were spending much of their time on routine FMD checks for the Ministry. FMD is an extremely infectious viral disease of cattle, sheep and pigs, causing a high fever followed by blistering of the mouth and feet. Most animals eventually recover but the economic and welfare effects of leaving the disease unchecked is massive. The actual mortality is low in adults at under 5% but higher in young stock.

In early March, all the cattle on a farm no more than two miles away from my home were slaughtered as they had contact with the initial Essex outbreak. The smell of disinfectant was strong enough to reach home. The disease was indeed awfully close. The next week the dog and cat congress was taking place in Birmingham and I attended a meeting trying to recruit vets to help with the massive problems with FMD overrunning British farms, especially in Cumbria.

I knew the practice could spare me so volunteered. I expected a call sending me to the north of England so was preparing myself for a bit of a drive. When the call came within a couple of days, I was told that I was needed at Dumfries. After some discussion I offered to fly to Glasgow from Gatwick, then hire a car and the Ministry of Agriculture (MAFF) voice on the phone agreed with the plan and I was on a plane a few days later – a Sunday. All the contingency plans and paperwork were describing infected premises but by mid-March with over 240 infected premises and rising it was more logical to talk of infected counties. The contiguous slaughter policy was brought in. This stated that all animals within two miles of an infected premises must be slaughtered. This was immediately clarified to mean sheep only. All the pigs, cattle and sheep on the infected premises were to be slaughtered but the contiguous cull was to act as a disease "firebreak".

So, I checked in at the guesthouse in Dumfries and the next morning went to Dumfries VI Centre. From there I was sent to the middle of the town where army groups were gathering with slaughter men, council workers and vets to make themselves into teams, and after poring over maps drove off on their designated killing spree. It all felt like an Einzatsgrupen genocide operation on the eastern front of WWII, until I saw tears in the eyes of several young squaddies who were badly traumatised by what they were about to do, probably because they had been part of these mass slaughter squads earlier in the month or because they had heard about them.

As nobody knew me and asked me to join their squad, I was told to go back to the VI Centre for the 11am briefing. At that meeting there was again much poring over a larger map of the region covering Cumbria, Glasgow, Dumfries and Stranraer. The meeting was mainly attended by vets on FMD patrol ahead of where the disease had got to. The Stranraer group of vets were saying, or rather Hugh their spokesman was saying, they felt the disease would be heading west towards them soon and because of the contiguous slaughter policy they were deprived of experienced vets and incredibly low on the required team numbers.

I was immediately asked if I would join them in Stranraer the next morning. I certainly did not fancy joining the army killing squads so willingly accepted. That left me that afternoon and I was given a black bag full of index cards and asked to deliver the record cards back to a farm just outside of Dumfries. As most of my drive from Glasgow the day before had been down the motorway, I had not noticed the lack of livestock but suddenly on the road out to the farm I passed three still burning pyres with recognisable cattle carcasses on them and noticed not a single grazing animal on the way to the dairy farm. I saw the sign swinging on the road telling me it was the home of the pedigree Guernsey dairy herd I was looking for. As I parked the car and went into the dairy, with my sad plastic bag, I was greeted by a member of the family. He told me he and his father had farmed there all his life and the initial herd was founded by his grandfather. His father was in the house still in shock after the slaughter of the herd the week before. It was tragic to see a dairy farmer standing on an empty farm, by an empty bulk milk tank and a spotless parlour just milking ghosts.

Rather than just hand over the black bag and run, which is what part of me wanted to do, I had to talk to this devastated man. I put my hand in the bag and saw the number 22 and all the clinical details of a wonderful five-year-old milker whose butterfat (BF) was high and last annual milk yield particularly good for the breed. It was obviously the right thing to do because the farmer was choking up and wanted to talk. He told me yes, she was a great cow and how his neighbour, also a dairy farmer, got the disease a couple of weeks ago and after killing that herd MAFF just decided to kill his. He knew it was inevitable but it still hurt to see perfectly healthy cows killed.

Because they were a closed pedigree herd, it was such a tragedy to lose such a wonderful genetic line. He said 22 was typical and no matter what compensation he got, a direct link with his grandfather's cows and his grandfather had been extinguished. I got the distinct impression that the officious approach of the authorities had not helped an obviously grieving family. I continued the conversation and he acknowledged it would have been worse for the herd to succumb to the disease which would have devastated him and his father. I certainly did not leave him happy, but I left him less miserable than when I arrived, and he seemed genuinely pleased to have his records back.

The next morning, I checked out of my digs. It was a one star "the door is locked at 10.30pm and you can borrow a key if you really are going to be any later but please be quiet if after 11", sort of place. I drove to Stranraer: it was 60 miles along the Ayr coast and suddenly after Ayr no more pyres and cattle and sheep grazing along the route.

If the vegans get their way the world will be a strange place.

I found the VI office and I introduced myself to the Divisional Veterinary Officer (DVO), the senior full-time MAFF vet in the area. He showed me around and introduced me to the local team that were in the office at the time. I then loaded my car with protective equipment and spent the rest of the afternoon looking at the patrol plans for the area over the next week or so and looking at a larger scale OS map of the region. Hugh and other members of his team then gradually returned from their patrols. I became aware there were two groups of vets and teams: clean ones looking for FMD and dirty ones dealing with the disease. After an hour, the only dirty vet in the area arrived after suitable disinfection and I met Simon, a recent graduate from Dublin whose home was in Belfast. He had been thrown in a very deep end. He briefed us on the latest encroachment in our area by the virus, telling us that day he had supervised the slaughter of a herd of a hundred dairy cows 50 miles east of Stranraer and certainly west of the contiguous sheep slaughter of the day before from Dumfries meant to protect our area.

We all stayed at the Castle Hotel in Stranraer which is now known as the North West Castle Hotel. It was a memorable stay with a great team with some highs and some very deep lows. The next day I went out on patrol checking about four flocks in the morning and four in the afternoon. It was easier to check if they were brought in to pens or barns but none of my flocks had any lesions or signs. That first day was typical of my first ten days in Stranraer: lots of fear but no sign of any problems. Dealing with the farmers was like my first days in farm practice. Lots of time to chat, lots of "while you are here can you look at this one", but always the underlying threat that disaster was heading in from the east.

As well as routine patrols, we also had to respond to calls where farmers were suspicious that their stock had the disease. Because the compensation price was going up, some farmers were looking to cash in on their flock or herd for the generous pay out, but most were not. As usual, most farmers were generous and kind as well as welcoming.

One of the characters I met dealing with his flock and a few head of cattle was a local farmer who had the most well-trained sheep or cattle working dogs and a couple of quad bikes. He and a mate could help with any unruly stock for a small fee and I certainly wrote his mobile down in my old Nokia as I had a feeling that would come in handy.

In my first week I was asked by Hugh to go and check a calf that was drooling. Hugh told me to take the paperwork declaring the premises infected and restricting the farm as I arrived. He obviously feared it might be FMD. As I got to the farm, I signed the Form A and issued it to the stockman. I then looked at the large beef suckler calf which was still with its mother. It was certainly drooling. Its temperature was normal and there were no foot lesions. One look in the great big calf's mouth confirmed the problem. His tongue was lacerated by his own lower incisor teeth. His mother had kicked at him when he forcefully sucked and bunted her by now tender udder. The tongue was badly bitten a third of the way down but not severed and would heal. It was not FMD. I checked his mother, including her udder, and again no sign of disease, including a normal temperature. I checked the rest of the herd and no sign of disease so I signed the farm release document Form B and gave a copy to the herdsman telling him to wean the calf as soon as it was over the immediate trauma and told him it would need a course of antibiotic and anti-inflammatory treatment.

When I got back to the office after routine on-farm sterilisation, I faxed the forms to Page Street in London. Within minutes the office phone rang for me and I was asked by an irate caller from Page Street: "By whose authority had I released the farm from its FMD restrictions?" I replied, "It was not FMD." "How do you know?" I explained how I knew. "How long have you been qualified?" he asked, and was a little taken aback when I replied, "27 years." "Dogs and cats, I suppose!" he stated. "No," I said, "I am from a mixed practice in Cranbrook, Kent." He repeated, "How do you know it was not FMD?" And I was told his superior would ring me back and to get ready to be sent home. I was flabbergasted but not sorry and when he got into the office, I told Hugh. "Well done," he said, "you have woken that lot up." I asked what he would have done. "Do not ask me," he replied, because he did not do things by the book.

About 8pm I got a phone call from Page Street on my mobile; the caller was charming: he asked a few questions and I explained. "Fantastic," he said, "You have done everything correctly and you are just the sort of person we need in the frontline, but you should not have released the farm after your examination without contacting us." "Why? The calf had been kicked?" "I know but we are only allowed to cull contiguous sheep and if we had wanted to kill the cattle herd your certification was perfect." "But it was not FMD." "It was until you issued the clearance certificate. You released the premises." I realised his point and it was a political one. "So, shall I pack my bag? Your colleague was adamant I should." "No," he repeated, "you are just the sort of chap we need there." And he put down the phone.

Later after supper over a drink I told Hugh and the others about the phone call and asked Hugh what he did that was different and not by the book. He told me he wrote the paperwork declaring the farm infected but did not give it to anyone. If something like my case, he ripped the form up after leaving the farm. "Only ever let Page Street agree to release. I told you to take the paperwork, not sign and issue it." When I questioned him as to why he did not tell me before, he said, in his broad Scottish accent, "'Cos that's not by the 'book'." From then on, we all did it Hugh's way.

Including when I was asked to go and check some sheep at Barrhill which was 30 miles away. The call came in about 5pm. Hugh laughed because I was asked by the DVO to go. When I asked why he was laughing, Hugh said because it is miles away and he did not fancy going himself at 5pm. I looked at the map and Barrhill was only 30 miles away, wondering why just a half-hour drive would get that reaction. I soon found out, or rather after an hour's drive down winding roads I found out. With my paperwork ready but not presented, I greeted the very enthusiastic family who were both excited and worried to be involved in the crisis. The call was for a few slobbering ewes and lambs on the farm. It was obvious on looking at the flock that many of them had Orf, a disease also called contagious pustular dermatitis, which is a viral infection transmissible to people. It is a self-limiting disease but can affect the ability of lambs to feed and suck from the ewes or graze if old enough. The sores are different to FMD, but blisters can form. The temperatures I checked were all normal and although one lamb did have blisters in its mouth, they were Orf blisters. I was convinced the flock just had Orf and told the family so. Advising them if the flock did survive the outbreak, Orf vaccination was available and "prevention was better than cure". The drive back to Stranraer took even longer in the dark and I had missed supper by the time I got back to the hotel. Hugh laughed as he presented me with a sandwich he had ordered for me. "Told you it was a long way to Barrhill."

The next day the DVO asked how I got on and I told him it was Orf. Hugh chuckled. Hugh and I had the last laugh as the office phone went again at 5pm that day with the same family asking for another visit. I offered to go again but the DVO said he would and set off. The next morning, I asked him what he thought. "Orf," he replied. "You were right." Hugh and I suppressed a laugh and I said, "It's a long way to Barrhill," sharing a knowing look with Hugh. "Yes, only 30 miles," the DVO commented, "but takes ages." I did not ask him if he issued the paperwork but suspect he too did it Hugh's way – not involving Page Street.

The disease was getting nearer, and Simon seemed to have a shorter commute to and from his various infected premises so much so that one night after ringing Page Street on some matter we joked that soon Page Street would have one of the new automated answering services: press A for contiguous slaughter of sheep, B for infected premises slaughter, and C to speak to someone.

The sad joke was on us because the following week it was us doing the slaughter of sheep in front of the outbreak. We went to sheep farms and met up with slaughter gangs: they killed the adult stock and the vets had to kill the lambs, trying to keep up with the gangs so the lambs were hardly separated from their mums when it was their turn. The adult stock was killed using humane captive bolts, but the lambs needed barbiturates. The best was a super concentrated form used for horses. If injected correctly in a lamb, death was very quick, and if into the heart instantaneous. Sadly, or the opposite, my cardiac skills meant I could keep up with the slaughtermen and the lambs were only separated from their mothers for a truly short time and the urgent high-pitched bleating of the lambs echoed by the deeper "baas" of their mothers was only brief.

It was a horrid, harrowing experience for all concerned and credit to the poor council workers who were not used to working with livestock but always made sure these family euthanasias went well with minimal delay between a group arriving and their despatch. It was on one of these farms that I got to know the best slaughter team and their leader whose number I also put into my phone memory for later use along with the good dogs and the quad bikes. I now fully understood why the groups that formed in Dumfries together on my first day were determined to stay together before going out on their contiguous culls and not have an unknown vet in their midst. They were bonded by the most awful situation.

The next day it was the same story and the day ending with a pile of adult sheep bodies to be buried and a horrible sad little mountain of lambs waiting patiently to be re-united with their mothers in a burial pit.

The third day was the toughest. Any doubts were gone. I knew I had killed more lambs in the last two days than I had saved in my whole veterinary career. I tried to cheer myself by thinking good job done but my heart broke when I saw the day's flock. They were a beautiful pedigree Border Leicester flock with their cute, characteristic Roman noses. Most of the ewes had twins. My first response was a professional one. I checked the name of the farm and the special map reference we were given to make sure we were in the correct place. Then emotion took over and I shed a quiet tear; luckily it was windy and blustery, and nobody noticed. The morning went well, and the refreshment truck arrived in the middle of the farm. I told him he should have waited at the gate. The driver reminded me we were not on an infected farm and he had not been on one. Not the point, I told him, making him disinfect himself before driving off.

After lunch, as we started to separate the lambs from the ewes, a council worker came up to my makeshift desk which was built of straw bales. He had half a dozen gorgeous lambs tucked under his arms. Three under each. He rang on a pretend bell and said, "Two o'clock appointment with Dr Shipman please." I laughed until tears ran down my face. I now really understood what was meant by gallows humour. As I despatched the poor little souls with the help of the council worker, we both still had tears in our eyes but were they tears of laughter? Harold Shipman had murdered perhaps 250 patients in his care and had the nickname "Dr Death". He committed suicide by hanging three years after FMD. I was also a Dr Death. Was a contiguous kill a genuine preventive medicine technique? I suppose it was if the animals saved from the disease outnumbered the animals killed making the "firebreak". I was asked if I wanted to go on another cull at 3.30pm when we finished but I turned my back on my day's little mountain, got in my car and drove back to the hotel. I went to my room and buried my head in the pillow and waited for the bar to open.

The next day there was no contiguous sheep kill and I was feeling much refreshed and in the office having coffee when Simon rang in for some help. He was on a farm where he was sure the cow he looked at had FMD. He had issued the paperwork but was having trouble getting a slaughter team and all the stock were scattered over several fields. Some had even broken into a neighbour's farmland by jumping a fence as he and the farmer rounded them up. My trusted Nokia mobile was just drying out so I could not ring any contacts immediately. I always tied a long rectal glove or plastic bag around it when on a farm, but the bag had leaked so before I went to the bar the night before I had dismantled it into its three components and the sim and put it near the radiator overnight. I had taken it to the office that morning but not yet reassembled it. I quickly pieced it together and put in the card. It immediately searched for a signal and with the DVO's permission rang my favourite slaughter gang's number and the farmer with the two quad bikes and two lovely collies. The latter told me his stock had been slaughtered the week before and he was dirty. I gave him my condolences and asked if he needed work. He said he did and told him to meet me at the farm gate. The slaughter gang were still clean, according to their leader, as they had just dealt with contiguous kills and agreed to meet me on the farm.

I rushed to the farm and told Simon what I had arranged. He was expecting the auctioneer any minute and showed me a cow in the crush. She had a little burst blister on the inside of the upper lip and no other symptoms. Not very spectacular, I said, are there any other cases? He told me most of the stock was out but three yearlings he had managed to get in were clear. Anyway, he said, Page Street have called it so the whole farm was going to be slaughtered. OK, I said: "Where is the farmer?" at which point an irate farmer came charging out of the house. So, a Scot was faced by a Northern Irishman and me. "Are you English?" he demanded. I said yes but my "Dad was Belgian," I quickly added as I saw his clenched fist as if that might save me.

He seemed to calm as if he noticed I had a southern English accent and had calculated I had come a long way and therefore deserved a little credit rather than the punch I think he first wanted to administer. "The cattle are all over the place. Is it foot-and-mouth?" I had to calm him down as he then shouted, "They won't even let my wife and kids on the farm. She has gone to her sister's." I told him I had got just the man to round up his cattle and to go back inside for a cup of tea. He was just about to argue when the slaughter team turned up. "Now there are enough of us to get the cattle in," I said, "You go in." He said he would join us when luckily the auctioneer turned up, so he had to go inside and value the herd and his sheep flock to obtain the compensation. It was a disaster trying to round up the cattle and more jumped into the neighbour's. Then I heard a honking at the end of the drive. The quad bikes had arrived. "The cavalry are here," I said to Simon, and rang the cavalry again on my perfectly functioning mobile. Soon the quad bikers and the dogs had got a yard full of cattle in for us and there was a chance to check some more in the run.

All seemed OK until we got to the last cow in the run, she had definite vesicles on her tongue that ruptured when Simon touched it. "That's a definite case," I murmured. "Shall we get started as the light will fade before we have finished," I asked. "No," said Simon, we must wait for the auctioneer. We were about ten miles from Stranraer and the disease had come all the way across from Dumfries and did not look like it would stop soon. An hour later the farmer came to the door, saw we were waiting and went back inside. He was driving a hard bargain with the auctioneer. We started to unload lights that were arriving and then a generator came. It was then that the auctioneer came out and said from a distance we could go ahead. Simon warned him he was now "dirty" having visited an infected premise and gave him advice not to visit another farm and get further information from MAFF.

We started to kill the cattle. The chief slaughterman was brilliant: he was almost like a horse whisperer. He would make a funny noise with his lips and the cows would move forward into the crush, then he waved his fingers in front of their face. Then suddenly "bang" with the captive bolt and their eye would go out. By which I mean on the "b" of bang I could see the pupil dilated and the cornea went from moist to bone dry. The beast was then quickly hobbled and dragged out using a tractor after pithing. Pithing is the destruction of the spinal cord by passing a flexible rod into the head wound down the spinal canal. There seemed no fear from the cattle behind, just curiosity. It is amazing considering how stressed they were coming into the yard that they seemed impatient for their turn. He almost called them in with his spooky fingers and lip-smacking sounds. The bull went in as quietly as the three cows before him. Then another bang and he went down. Two more cows and suddenly the farmer appeared with his fists clenched again, and he was heading straight for the cattle whisperer. I stepped between them, which was stupid because both were strong enough to look after themselves, and I could smell the whisky. "You've killed my bull," the farmer said, trying and succeeding in pushing me aside. At which point Simon called out "Look at this." I took the farmer by the arm over to the bull's carcass as Simon lifted his lips and pulled out his tongue. The mouth was covered in vesicles at all stages – forming, ruptured and healing. "Billy was riddled with it," I shouted above the nearby tractor noise. This calmed the farmer, and he went back in doors hopefully not having more whisky, leaving us to continue our sad job.

We worked under floodlights until 2am and all the cattle were killed, leaving just the sheep. It was sensibly decided to call it a night as despite the floodlights the visibility was not that good. We aimed to start again at 10am but suddenly a very drunk farmer came out of the house again ready to punch anyone that stood in his way. "What do you mean leave the sheep?" I again stepped up and said, "I have heard from other farmers that when the whole farm's livestock is taken, that the silence in the morning is horrid. At least you will hear the sheep when you wake up in the morning." He burst into tears and put his arms around me. I smelt the whisky on his breath stronger than earlier and felt his whiskers on my face as he gave me a big man hug and then went back in the house.

We started again the next day at ten and the farmer helped us get the sheep in and, although he was more than a little hungover, behaved extremely pleasantly after his first night on his own since the day he got married.

I was now a dirty vet and was only allowed onto highly suspect farms. Later that afternoon I was called by a colleague to attend a farm near the village of Glaserton, Whithorn. Little did I realise this was the village a lady had barricaded herself in her house with five sheep to prevent them being culled by the firebreak scheme. A colleague had called me because she had been asked to check a cow but had found no real sign of FMD but was suspicious. When I arrived, I saw she was a suckler so asked where her calf was. "He's a big bull calf and still out in the field," the stockman told us. We jumped in his Land

Rover and after a little chasing caught the calf. It had a temperature of 110 degrees F (43.3C). I had seen calves with pneumonia with ones as high as 106 but never this high. Even allowing for the chase, that was outrageous. The only answer was issuing the form that the premises might have FMD. After checking the rest of the stock, we rang Page Street and told them of the suspect cow and calf, and they said as it was now 6pm to re-visit in the morning and they would get everything ready to cull the herd if there were more signs. We went back to the farm next morning at 6am and both cow and calf had classic FMD and so too did a stable full of young calves elsewhere on the yard.

I had to supervise the slaughter and by the afternoon three giant pyres with dead cattle on were burning in the field we had chased the calf in just the day before. One of the tractor drivers putting a cow carcass on the pyre pointed to a house down the hill telling me the lady had lost her case in the Edinburgh high court and the sheep would be culled. There was no chance of an appeal with pyres burning within sight of her home.

My month on FMD duty finished the following day and like the previous four weeks the weather was lovely when I said goodbye and got in my car to drive to Glasgow and get my flight home. Not one grazing animal the whole trip. On the train ride home from Gatwick it was like getting home from a holiday – but who returns from holiday with a suitcase full of neatly laundered almost sterilised clothes and nightmare memories.

The Netherlands had controlled their outbreak with vaccination, could we have done the same? Probably not, but vaccination will almost certainly be used to control any future outbreak in the UK.

22

THE DARK SIDE

Austen, a long-standing friend of mine who owned his own practice for many years, has always referred to vets who work in the pharmaceutical and corporate side of the industry as working for the dark side. I never thought I would get involved with this, but I did. After returning from FMD duty, it took the rest of the year for things to settle down and I got several teaching contracts from different veterinary education companies, lecturing in both dentistry and cardiology. I always enjoyed those odd days away from the practice somewhere in the country teaching vets and trying to impart some of my knowledge and experience. Within practice I was always keen to spot disease early and once spotted finding out what could be done to slow or reverse the disease.

As I have said earlier, I believe correct nutrition is a key to a long, healthy life and sad to say American pet food manufacturers were ahead of the game. When I first got to Cranbrook there was a therapeutic diet available for dogs with renal disease and we certainly used it. Then along came a complete range from America with therapeutic diets for both dogs and cats for a range of diseases including heart, liver, kidney, obesity and diabetes. We were all very well trained in their use by the company with lots of evening lectures and there was soon no doubt in my mind that these diets prolonged life. The adage "You are what you eat" is so true: it means that it is important to eat good food to be healthy and fit and, furthermore, when health problems such as obesity, diabetes, renal, heart, liver, dental or skin problems come along, then dietary modifications may help control those diseases.

For example, pets with renal disease seem to benefit from control of the level of protein in the diet. Too high and of poor quality means the kidneys must work harder. Similarly, salt levels are important; many proprietary pet foods contain too much, especially in the face of background renal, cardiac or hepatic problems.

In April 1991, a new giant petfood manufacturer wanted a share of the pet health food "pie", if that is the right word. They were trying to get our wholesaler to stock their products but before commitment the wholesaler suggested they contact a neighbouring practitioner, Dr Jackson of Sevenoaks, and me to sound out what we thought of their products. They went one better and invited us to their headquarters in St Louis. We duly flew out, but it was a typical show and tell with senior management within the giant company juggling major projects but not focusing fully on any and certainly not on the prescription diet market.

They wanted to launch a renal diet for dogs but were unaware of the massive problem renal disease was in cats. They were playing catch-up very badly because during a visit to their research cattery where their diets were trialled for normal healthy cats, we asked, "What happens to any cats showing signs of renal disease?" and were told they were euthanased, which did not bode well for that company working on a renal diet for cats. When we tried to schedule a meeting to discuss our findings, the "big cheese" was already pre-occupied with the launch of a human tea cake which he invited us to try – and jolly nice they were too – but we were certainly not going to provide the positive feedback to our wholesaler that either party wanted.

As far as the diets for healthy dogs and cats were concerned, the St Louis-based company was top notch with a diet for each life stage but nowhere near the prescription diet market. The best thing about the trip was a ride within the St Louis landmark, the 630-foot Gateway Arch, and a baseball match between the St Louis Cardinals and the Braves.

When we got back to the UK, we were shown the new life-cycle range from our usual supplier. Believe it or not, at the time in the

UK it was not possible to buy a diet specifically for a puppy or an elder dog: all pet foods were one size fits all. It was also not possible to buy a diet suitable for a giant dog like a Great Dane or a toy dog like a Chihuahua. This all changed in the nineties, but I would still argue that pet nutrition has a long way to go with the recent craze for raw meaty bone diets for dogs. The propaganda talks of a reduction of allergies and increased palatability but there is no doubt these are unbalanced diets with remarkably high protein (hence the palatability) with the potential for whole bones to cause problems, but the biggest threat to human and dog health is the bacteria potentially present in raw food including *Salmonella, E. coli* and *Campylobacter*. The first step to health must be to feed a healthy, balanced diet and then when there is a health problem feed a diet that helps manage that disease.

I was then invited by a vaccine manufacturer to speak at the launch of their new cat vaccine in September 1999. It was a multivalent all-in-one syringe vaccine that covered all seven preventable cat diseases: the two sorts of flu, chlamydia an infectious conjunctivitis, panleucopaenia and leukaemia. Not surprisingly it was called "Pentofel". At last, we could protect our cat patients against all these diseases in one injection. I had good contacts with the company for years but got on particularly well with the company vet Ben. He had been in practice in East Sussex and often referred both dental and cardiac patients to me.

He approached me and asked if I would be one of the speakers at the product launch. This took place over a week at venues in London, Bristol, Manchester and Edinburgh. I had to talk mainly about my practice's experience of using a chlamydial vaccination programme to reduce the infectious conjunctivitis cases in our cat patients. We had used a vaccine against it since one was launched by the same company nearly a decade before. I found that as a common disease it could and should be prevented. Others felt that a simple infectious conjunctivitis was better treated with antibiotics rather than prevented by vaccination. I could never see the logic of this view. The London meeting went well – it should have done as it was held in Simpson's-in-the-Strand – and two days later I was addressing a large meeting in Bristol. The cat leukaemia virus part of the talk was given by an American vet, Arne, who worked for the company and he spoke eloquently about how many more cats' lives could be saved from this immuno-compromising disease if only a higher percentage of our pet cats were vaccinated against it.

It would be fair to say that at the time half of cat owners bringing cats to practices in the UK were not offered protection against this preventable fatal disease. My year mate Tim, who was now a lecturer at Bristol University vet school, spoke about cat flu viruses. Vaccination against these viruses was only now being used regularly in UK practices but like our practice, uptake for cat vaccination was low – under 50% amongst our clients and our percentage was far higher than many. A few days later and Ben collected me from home, and he drove us up to Manchester for the launch meeting. It went well with the same speakers giving the same presentations. The next morning Ben drove me up to Edinburgh.

Ben was a good if fast driver but often had to field phone calls regarding technical enquiries for the company's other products. This was fine by me except that he did not seem to slow down during these calls over the few days he drove me. The final straw was when he decided to take the more scenic route to Edinburgh, leaving the motorway after Carlisle and driving along the tortuous but picturesque roads through the glens. Ben was a smoker at the time, and he managed to drive and negotiate the bendy road very well whilst having a cigarette. However, a technical query during a cigarette and a signal dropping out was a little too much for me as he was steering with his knees, smoking his cigarette, and redialling a number on his mobile.

I suggested he pull over and park, finish his cigarette and deal with the phone call. "Jeepers, It's like 'Driving Miss Daisy'," he said, referencing the recent popular film where an elderly southern American Jewish lady has an African American chauffeur. We both laughed but he did from then on limit his multi-tasking to just smoking and driving or talking hands-free and driving but never again steering with his knees.

The talk in Edinburgh went particularly well but I was perhaps a little shocked when the local company representative, Bryan, went to each attending practitioner during the meal and did not let them continue their meal until he had got an order. Not surprisingly, hopefully for the benefits, not the Scottish hard sell, Pentofel went on to be the leading cat vaccine for many years. Bryan went on to be UK sales director of another leading vaccine company.

Despite the success of dog and cat vaccination programmes, there was always opposition from anti-vaccinators both within the medical professions and outside of them. The claim that MMR vaccination caused human autism was around for years but came to a head in 1998 when a now discredited paper was published in *The Lancet* that year and its author Andrew Wakefield became popular. The widely publicised debate led to a crash in the number of kids vaccinated and as an inevitable spin-off veterinary vaccination uptake also declined. Similar anti-vaccination reports were aimed at dog and cat vaccination programmes. There was and is a feeling in some quarters that over-vaccination was occurring. A lot of this criticism came from North America and because of trying to defend their vaccines in the USA I was invited by Ben's company to join him at a Feline Medicine Conference in Steamboat Springs near Denver in Colorado during the winter of 2002. A key speaker at that conference was a Dr Lapin who had been trying unsuccessfully to prove in his research that a cell culture used in feline vaccine manufacture was a cause of cat renal failure.

The vaccine company wanted to host an evening meeting giving the counter-argument to some of the anti-vaccinators. I was one of the speakers at that meeting. Another was the world authority on a cat neck cancer that was said to be caused by vaccination. The anti-group even gave it the name cat vaccine sarcoma. I have seen three cases, one admittedly was vaccinated every year, the second had never had any injection at all and the third had once had an injection of penicillin. The view of the expert veterinary epidemiologist Phillip was that there was no proven correlation between vaccination and the neck skin cancer.

I attended Dr Lapin's lecture and in his most emotive anti-vaccination stance invited any member of the audience to go onto his stage and be injected with "a foreign protein". I immediately put my hand up and volunteered. When he asked me, "Why would I do that?" I replied, "Because I have my flu inoculation every year and wasn't that a foreign protein?"

There is still a movement against vaccination, campaigning against vaccines regarded as non-core as if some diseases are unimportant and should just be tolerated. Sadly, I think that some of the individuals promoting these views are just self-promoting. Even now the World Small Animal Veterinary Association (WSAVA) argues against "needless vaccination, preferring in-house antibody tests and risk assessments" almost as if vaccines can cause real harm. Adverse effects do happen, extremely rarely and, in my experience, so rarely that the benefits far outweigh these minor side effects which are usually easily treated.

A group of drugs called ACE inhibitors (ACEI) are used in human medicine to control symptoms and the damage caused by cardiac disease, high blood pressure and kidney disease. These drugs had been quickly used for renal disease in cats and heart disease in dogs but remained unlicensed for heart disease in cats and renal disease in dogs. Amber was a nine-month-old boxer puppy when she started showing signs of renal (kidney) failure. It had been established for several years that special low salt, lower protein high B vitamin diets were useful in both dogs and cats with kidney disease and she was on this but what else could be done to help her? The first step was to investigate the cause of her renal disease more thoroughly. Her owner wanted her spayed as Amber felt worse after being in season and went completely off food so it was agreed to get a set of kidney biopsies at the same time as the spay op.

These were taken and proved which type of renal disease she had but her blood tests were looking worse and renal transplantation is not an option in dogs. It was agreed to use ACE inhibitor drugs, and these helped Amber to live until she was just over 11 years old – a normal life span – and until the end she had a great quality of life.

What about the use of this drug in heart disease in both dogs and cats? The commonest heart disease in dogs is mitral valve disease (MVD) in which the valve degenerates over time because of protein material being deposited in it and causing thickening, degeneration and the valve closes less efficiently. This valve is on the left side of the heart between the two chambers and as it starts to leak, every heartbeat blood goes back up into the top chamber, the atrium, from the ventricle instead of out through the aorta. As the disease progresses, the atrium increases in size and eventually congestive heart failure occurs. ACE inhibitor drugs were licensed and proven to be useful in treating this disease. The big debate was how early in the disease was the drug useful.

I was then approached during one of the dog and cat conferences in Birmingham by Graeme, a chap I knew who worked for the main manufacturer of the ACEI, because the sales of their drug were crashing due to the launch of a new heart drug. All the vets in practice were dropping their use of ACEI and switching to the new drug. All the veterinary cardiologists believed both drugs had a place in treatment but did not agree which drug was to be used first or when during the battle against MVD they should be used along with other available drugs. There was also the issue of which ACEI was best, as there were several available.

As a result, I signed a contract with the ACEI company to go out on the road three days a week, leaving me two days a week in the practice and my share of the weekend rota.

My aim was to improve the approach of veterinary general practitioners to cardiac disease and the company's approach was to stop and reverse their crashing ACEI sales. Was this selling out to the dark side? I believed the standard of cardiac care amongst my colleagues could be lifted and lives saved. This might level the balance for the lives I had taken during FMD.

The format was standard. I would set off on a train from my local station and spend three days on the road with one of the drug company's representatives. We would go into practices in the morning, afternoon or lunchtime and then hold a meeting in hotels of an evening. The talk was everything from one-on-one during the day to large multi-practice groups in the evening. I would often discuss individual cardiac cases on PowerPoint, sometimes seeing the practice's own cardiac cases run ECG and echoes (ultrasound of hearts) and then logically help them with therapy.

I went all over England, Scotland, Wales and Northern Ireland, including a memorable couple of trips to the Republic with a well-attended meeting in Dublin. I got several exceedingly kind feedback comments but the most memorable one from a Dublin vet who said: "I go to a lot of these evening meetings and say to myself, 'One day I will do that in my practice', and sadly never do. What you have told me tonight about investigating and treating my heart cases I will do from tomorrow."

I will never forget one of the area managers from the south-west, James, who was very hands-on and spent a lot of time on the road warning me: "Beware of when you pull in the drive at home and the dog barks at you − it means you have been away too long."

I laughed but within the year it happened.

Apart from positive feedback from the vets and their practices, how could it be proven that I was making a difference with the road tour? The ACEI sales were improving but was that just thanks to my talks or not?

The answer was shown using sales figures from the Isle of Wight. I did a series of talks on the island and the quarterly sales figures for ACEI went up 60% − no wonder I was given another contract the following year. Another less pleasant sign was that I got a solicitor's letter from the manufacturer of the other heart drug accusing me of maligning their product. This was false. I had been to the launch of their new drug in Germany and used a large amount of it, but not as the only drug I used. I immediately contacted the company with the sales figures for their drug in my practice and argued my case. Consequently, if I mentioned their drug in my talks, which I did, I could not mention the trade name, only the active drug − pimobendan. That was fine by me.

After a negotiation period I got another contract from the company. This one also included a bonus percentage if the sales improved. To get to the area I was needed it often meant a 5am train to London, then on to where I was headed – Manchester, Bristol, Cardiff or wherever. Often it meant flights from Gatwick and one day I even commuted to Inverness and back in a day to help train a practice with ECG and echo.

The PowerPoint presentations were often of my referred or in-house patients at the time. One of these was Digby, a Cavalier King Charles spaniel born in 1992, and as a five-year-old he had a loud mitral valve murmur due to MVD. He had x-ray and ECG changes and was put on ACEI. He was also unwilling to exercise but how do you tell with a lazy spaniel if he has poor exercise tolerance? According to his owner, it improved on the therapy. The debate is interesting as to when treatment should start but he lived to be 12 years old and was on both the accepted heart drugs when he went into classic congestive heart failure at 11 years of age, then sadly died suddenly, at which time he was also on diuretics.

The big question was always: would any drugs really help early in cardiac disease before and if so which ones?

My cardiac colleague Chris, who worked in Canterbury, put it succinctly, "Dogs need ACEI the week before they go into congestive heart failure." It is obviously impossible to know that time but a case of sooner rather than later and there is much evidence in humans for early use.

Then there was a breakthrough: an American cardiologist published a paper showing a benefit of longer life in dogs treated with ACEI, but many cardiologists dismissed the paper and found scientific holes in it, leaving many dogs untreated until they were actually in heart failure.

My advocacy of ACEI was made more difficult by the publication of a paper showing that if just one of the two drugs was used, ACEI did not do so well. Interesting that neither company wanted to fund the research: we all suspected that together the two drugs worked better than either alone – typical of the so-called dark side. Amazingly, for all my trips around the British Isles, I only did a few presentations in my home county of Kent.

The second contract was up, and I was interested to hear from sales data obtained from the wholesalers that the sales of ACEI for the company were up by 6%. That would mean a handsome bonus, not for me personally but the practice as all the consulting fees were paid to the partnership.

I could not have been more mistaken. Apparently, no bonus was due because by the time the costs of my consultancy and the costs of the subsidised ECG machines that had been given to practices were considered, the increased sales profits were lost. Not that the contract made this clear, but I settled for a further three-month contract rather than litigation.

The following year another company offered me a six-lecture tour discussing their drug which was a combination of the same ACEI and a mild diuretic type of drug which had a cardio-protective effect demonstrated in both dogs and man. One of the six venues was the Isle of Wight and the wheel turned full circle to be back there. Recently there have been papers which prove the drug that caused the crash in ACEI sales has a definite benefit in canine cardiac disease before the onset of CHF, so now there is no reason not to treat heart disease early and the Steele-Bodger middle group is now so much larger than in 1973.

Another cardiac disease I regularly discussed was cardiomyopathy. Dogs commonly get the dilated form (DCM) and cats the hypertrophic thickening form (HCM), but the dilated form does occur rarely in the cat and the hypertrophic form rarely in the dog. Just as mitral valve disease (MVD) is a disease of little dogs, DCM is a disease of larger breed dogs. Interestingly, Cocker spaniels can get either disease. Walbrook-Bear was a Newfoundland born in May 1997. When he was just four years of age, he was unable to exercise, was thirsty, off food and lost weight. He had fluid in his abdomen and a weak pulse with an obvious heart rhythm disturbance. ECG showed he had slow rate atrial fibrillation where the top chambers of the heart are not beating properly, bombarding his lower ventricles with impulses causing an ECG change but not at the fast rate usual for these cases, suggesting his heart muscle was extremely sick.

Heart scan on ultrasound showed how weak and thin his heart muscle was, typical of DCM. The ultrasound also showed fluid in his abdomen building up because of his heart failure. Treatment involved draining 4.5 litres of fluid from his abdomen, then using diuretics and heart drugs including both ACEI and pimobendan when it became available. Approximately once or twice a year the fluid would build up and often need drainage and then extra diuretic types added or doses adjusted; by August 2006 he was on over ten different drugs, luckily some of them were available as combinations, so he only needed six tablets night and morning. As his owners knew he was so poorly when Walbrook-Bear was first diagnosed, they went and got another younger Newfoundland dog who lived to be seven years old when he died of bone cancer, so amazingly Walbrook-Bear outlived his replacement, finally dying a year later.

23

ANIMAL HOSPITAL FOR SALE

When I finished my last drug company contract, my wife Sandra said, "Now you can sort out the practice!" Little did I realise what a profound statement that was. Just before I joined the practice in 1976, they had given up their hospital status and it had always been my ambition to regain this as we were a founder practice in the British Veterinary Hospitals Association (BVHA) group.

The public do not realise the standard of care hoops needed to gain this status and how not having it is an easier option. Cranbrook originally had it but gave up hospital status when Tim Heeley retired from the partnership just before I joined. He was an eye specialist; a qualification Larry also went on to acquire. I went to a meeting in 2000 and the chairman Simon introduced me as from Cranbrook, "The Harley Street of Kent", which was very flattering but did show the standard of our practice perhaps better than the title of hospital.

The partnership comings and goings since I joined were a bit like the six wives of Henry VIII, but instead of "divorced, beheaded, died, divorced, beheaded, survived" was more like "divorced, retired, died, retired, retired, beheaded, survived". Mel retired because of divorce, Eric retired, Larry died, Doug retired, Lawrence retired, Duncan beheaded whist I survived in the practice. Larry had died after a very brief illness from cancer; Lawrence after getting his cardiac qualification under me wanted to move on despite thinking he wanted to settle and accepted a partnership, and Duncan left the practice after breaking the partnership agreement. This left me as the last man standing and sole owner of the practice.

To run the practice and acquire my coveted hospital status, I knew I needed help. So I employed as clinical director an old friend and colleague, Mike. This gave the practice a distinct uplift and we obtained hospital status again the following year. Then I employed Hugh, a local farm and equine practitioner, as large animal clinical director looking after the horses, cattle and sheep, allowing Mike to concentrate his powers as small animal clinical director.

The same year I employed my daughter Rhianna as a receptionist. She had finished school and a college

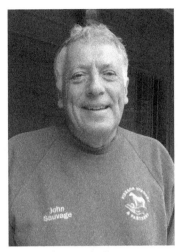

The author ready for action

course and was working shifts at a local pub, not fancying going to university. The landlord confirmed to me, as if I needed reminding but perhaps I did, what a hard worker she was and said what a wonderful telephone manner she had, so I offered her a receptionist's job. It was amazing how well Rhi took over the day-to-day management of the practice, almost instinctively knowing how I wanted the practice to run as if all those years of listening to me discussing the practice with her mother had been absorbed and she just thrived on more and more responsibility. She also carried out some of her own innovative ideas and improved client and patient care.

Within the year she was practice manager in all but name and a short time after that given the title officially. She was given the title on one proviso: that she studied for an external degree in business studies, which she did, being awarded a BA(Hons) with the Open University in 2018.

In the summer of 2016, I was called by my neighbour who years before had been a dairy client but now had a lovely, retired racehorse Apollo; he had won a single race at Lingfield in 2004 – his career as a novice. Then like so many ex-racers he fell through the net and ended up with my neighbour. He was now seventeen and had collapsed the day before. He was thin and underweight. I checked him and felt he was mainly undernourished with no evidence of dental or other digestive problems.

I was assured he was regularly wormed and on good hay and concentrates as well as grazing. I advised increasing his feeding plane dramatically as the summer progressed and I wormed him. I checked him again a month later and wormed him again. This time Sandra came with me. As he was thinner and weaker than on my first visit, I asked again what feed he was on. I was told the make of concentrate but when I asked to see the actual food was shown an empty bag and told another supply would be delivered shortly.

My wife offered to take over his feeding and very quickly went back with food concentrate and hay. It was obvious to both of us that Apollo was being neglected. Within a week Apollo was signed over to our care, a stable built, and he was grazing our home fields; within months he put on weight and was fit enough to be ridden again. His legs were not brilliant, but he soon enjoyed a little hack around our local bridleway. The following year his legs had deteriorated to such a level that he was retired from riding but as the winter of 2017 progressed, he became weaker and caste on several occasions and was unable to rise without assistance. He was by this time on multiple therapies including NSAIDs. One night In December the worst happened, and he went down in his stable and we made the tough decision to say goodbye. Over my career I have euthanased many horses, but Apollo was such a giant, kind fellow it was so hard to do without shedding a tear. He was down with his head lifting but completely unable to stand. His jugular vein was easily found, and a massive dose of barbiturate quickly administered, and Apollo laid his head down and peacefully stopped breathing. A stethoscope test proved his giant heart had stopped. The next day the local animal crematorium sympathetically collected him, and his ashes are still in our possession. This year, a rocking horse made by Stevenson Brothers of Bethersden and named Apollo, with his original reins, was alongside the Christmas tree for Penelope.

The hospital was busy and the business thriving. I began to get regular interest from corporate buyers and rebuffed their offers. I was not getting any younger, so eventually I signed a non-disclosure agreement with one and seriously negotiated with them, pending an offer. Finally, the offer came in but was not attractive and another corporate company made a more serious offer, and all was progressing towards a sale. A price was agreed and a completion date targeted. Only within three weeks of the sale date the company drastically reduced the offer, thinking I would accept a different deal now they sensed I was winding down to retirement. I declined the lower offer and went back to work, assuming I would carry on for another year or two. They were interesting times as good, experienced vets were getting hard to find and many only wanted to locum and worse still not cover out of hours with no farm or equine work. Leaving more and more to me at a time when I needed to do less.

This meant that for nearly a year I did more than my share of night duties, often all the farm and equine work as well as my cardiac and dental in-house and referral cases. It was just like a reprise of my first year in practice: I did a cattle calving, some sheep work including a caesarean, a horse colic case and a memorable uterine prolapse on a great big Charolais cow.

The prolapse of the uterus was a spectacular reminder of the college president's third group that you cannot help. The farmer was a long-standing client at a local farm in Cranbrook. It was a Saturday morning about 6am when I was called. The cow had calved, probably unsupervised, and then continued straining and instead of just the afterbirth passing the whole uterus had been pushed out.

Over the course of my career, I had successfully replaced dozens, but a lot depends on how long the prolapse had been out, causing it to swell and get damaged by being dragged behind the cow. I spent an hour trying to replace it. This involved washing the inside-out organ and trying to feed it back inside the cow using a plastic sack to suspend it and then inch by inch push it back after a spinal epidural to stop the cow straining. I never managed to get more than half in before the whole 35kg engorged organ fell out again. Rather than give up, I decided I needed help so rang a nearby cattle-only practice for support.

I returned to my Saturday morning surgery waiting for their duty vet to either drop by the surgery or go direct to the farm. A young, strong Irish vet arrived and was happy to go to the farm alone. She was noticeably confident the offending organ would soon be replaced but rang half an hour later needing my help. We both spent a further hour trying but never got more than a quarter of the now very bruised uterus back into the cow. It was obvious we had to give up and I then with the farmer's agreement shot the cow. You certainly cannot win them all but that was the first cow prolapse uterus I had failed to return – and the same for the vet who came to help me. Interestingly, after admitting failure, the destruction of the cow was left to me, suggesting how disappointed we both were. Another visit I collected was a farrowing at the Swattenden Centre in Cranbrook. It was a saddleback and she had produced two live piglets, then had complete womb inertia. Upon Internal examination a piglet could be felt so I pulled it out, with another behind. No others could be felt but as I described previously in a farrowing the weight of the womb can give the impression of more to come – but no more were within reach. A large dose of oxytocin produced two more piglets – a total of six so far. Regular doses of oxytocin left with the stockman meant she had a total litter of ten live little saddleback piglets by the next day when I checked her, but one had been born dead, making a litter size of eleven. During the check, her milk was coming well with no sign of the common post-farrowing mastitis/metritis syndrome in which infection strikes the womb and breast tissue after a prolonged farrowing.

At one of the calvings that year I took Sandra along for old time's sake, this time with a young, strong and fit Jake to pull on the calving ropes. The classic "first catch your patient" scenario also happened at Overbridge Farm in Marden with a lovely yearling bullock with an electric fence hook wedged under her eyelid. Each time we got her in the cattle run and crush on her own or with other members of the group, the farmer failed to shut the crush door and she alone or with other members of her gang escaped and then jumped back into the field. Just as I was wishing my old boss in Gloucestershire had lectured and trained the farmer, or my quad bike team would come and rescue us, we got the group in from the field one more time and in the melee in the race leading to the crush the hook was dislodged. When her neck was finally trapped in the crush with the door closed at last, I only had to apply some ointment to her sore eyelid and the job was done.

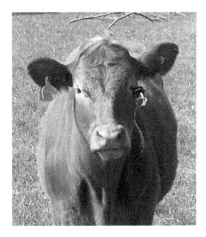

A yearling bullock with an electric fence hook caught under its eyelid. It was easily removed once the animal had been caught

Finally came an offer I could not refuse to buy the practice and the sale went through within six months of the offer. I was offered a year's work in the practice, but it was obviously time to leave.

So, after 43 years at Cranbrook, it was time to walk out for the last time. The practice had been my long-term mistress but at last the affair was over and I could go back to my wife. My daughter was due to go on maternity leave later that summer, but a premature labour meant that she left shortly after me, never to return to work there. Penny's early unannounced arrival takes me back to the beginning of this story as she was also in a hurry to get into this world. The whole family was camping in one of our fields on our farm. I had finally left the practice the month before and a very pregnant Rhi joined us for the Wednesday evening. Her baby was due in July and as she was a little uncomfortable a check scan had been booked for the following Saturday. Penny had other ideas and Rhi started getting severe stomach cramps on the Friday and was admitted to hospital on that day for an emergency caesarean.

My wife and her sister rushed to the hospital and witnessed the baby being pushed in an incubator from theatre towards the premature babies' intensive care wing. By the time I got to the hospital there was a rumour that Rhi was haemorrhaging from her liver and having a blood transfusion, but this was incorrect; the facts were that during the caesarean there was some abdominal bleeding from the womb that had probably caused the abdominal pain and early labour and this blood pooled near her liver.

After waking from her general anaesthetic and getting her transfusion, we could see our daughter along with her husband and his parents and she was recovering well. Mother and daughter were in hospital for a week together and then Penny was kept in the intensive baby unit for another month and finally released home near her mother's official due date.

EPILOGUE

The answer to the question "How did I get to where I am now?" is threefold. First and foremost is education. I added to my veterinary degree by studying O level and then A level political history at night school, and followed this up with an external degree with the Open University gaining an Upper Second Batchelor of Arts Honours degree in mainly history by studying whilst in practice between 1978 and 1987. I went on to gain a Certificate in Cardiology from the RCVS in 1989.

The other important physical and financial reason for getting where I am now is in real life's game of monopoly; whilst never owning hotels like my friend Chris, I have always when possible climbed up the property ladder both for my home and the practice. Initially, my little cottage in Sutton Valence, then the house attached to the Marden surgery between 1980 and 1985 and afterwards a rural property in Headcorn next to Graham's farm. In March 1985 I sold that and went to view a lovely cottage just outside the village of Collier Street; my offer was accepted on the basis that being a vet I would look after and treat the owner's daughter's old pony kept in a stable and field at the property, as the family felt the pony could not be moved. The deal was delayed as they were looking to get the lease on a pub.

Meanwhile, between March and September property prices did yet another of those "mad increases" that the bank manager in Maidstone predicted would never happen again after 1968. In late September, the expected call came from the vendor. He began the conversation: "We have got our pub and I am terribly sorry to have to inform you..." "Oh no," I thought, here comes the price re-negotiation. He continued,

"But my daughter wants to take our old pony." The deal went through at the original price and the old pony moved out with the owners, leaving me a large field and stable on which Sandra and I kept and fattened several head of cattle including three lovely Herefords which, when sold as stores for further fattening, got a special mention in the auctioneer's report.

Our next and final well-timed property move was to our farm in Egerton in 1999. It came complete with 23 acres of grazing land let to a neighbouring dairy farmer and the house needed massive renovation, but was worth it because the cottage in Collier Street sold well as so commutable to London whereas the Egerton Farm was a much further commute and therefore at the time an affordable price. My financial adviser, David, agreed to the purchase of the property if it could be sold as part of my pension. I agreed at the time but the only way I am leaving this home now is feet first.

I was also fortunate in other property deals. Firstly, on buying my partnership it came with the surgery freehold at Marden and a very long-term leasehold at the Headcorn Surgery; then in 1998 I helped the partnership negotiate the purchase of the Cranbrook premises from the family of the partner who retired when I joined the practice.

Whenever I wanted the partnership to buy property so our associate vets could live in them, this was overruled with David asking whether we were property investors or vets? For years, the practice paid rents to third-party landlords until at last as sole owner in 2011 I got my way and bought a little house in Cranbrook as vet assistant accommodation. Larry had always said we make more money on our homes in the beautiful Weald of Kent than we ever make vetting and that was so true. Kent really is the Garden of England and a main gateway to this "sceptred isle". The property I owned also helped secure the finance I needed from the banks to modernise and get the practice into the 21st century.

The final answer to the question, how did I get here from the little flat in Streatham to a lovely farmhouse in Kent, is luck. Luck firstly in having parents who allowed and encouraged me to start on my journey without spoiling me, albeit without a private education or an inheritance, and eventually finding that beautiful wife and everything coming together when it all seemed to be falling apart and could have gone so wrong without her firm support.

A recurring theme behind this story is my belief that the middle group of the triage can be expanded, more animals can be saved and the quality of their lives improved, with their longevity increased by good modern surgery and medicine. This can also be brought about by continuing improvements in preventive medicine techniques such as nutrition and vaccination.

As I said above, the badger debate continues but the government has planned a cattle TB vaccination programme by 2025 and a supplementary badger vaccination scheme in areas that have completed badger culls as an alternative to further culling. A third preventive way is to improve the genetic make-up of our patients by only breeding from good clean stock.

The dog hip scheme was in its infancy when I qualified, trying to remove the blight of dogs with bad hips, but now there are many joint, heart and eye schemes for breeding dogs, including DNA tests to try and eliminate these inherited diseases. I still see several breeding dogs a month to check that they are free from signs of heart disease, so their yet unborn puppies are free of congenital heart disease.

One of the most success-ful schemes I have been involved in since it started is the Boxer Heart Scheme. This involves listening to their hearts for murmurs and only allowing breeding from those cleared by a veterinary cardiologist.

This scheme has almost

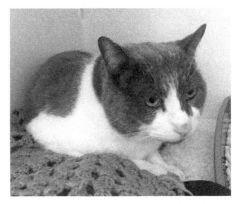

Blue, a 14-year-old cat with "gallop" heart rhythm

eliminated aortic stenosis from the breed, a disease where the exit from the heart to the aorta is congenitally constricted, blocking easy blood flow.

I also still see several heart cases at a local practice in Headcorn and one in Hastings at Vets4 Pets, part of the Pets at Home group. Just recently, with full Covid precautions, I went to Hastings at the request of the principal vet, Dan, to see Blue, a charming fourteen-year-old cat belonging to one of his nurses, Nicky. Blue had been seen the day before by Dan and his team with severe life-threatening breathing difficulties. Tests showed both chest cavity fluid (pleural) as well as fluid around his heart in the pericardial cavity. He is a lovely grey and white cat and when I examined him he was already much better than the previous day, thanks to the lifesaving diuretic treatment given. He was no longer open-mouthed breathing, but his breathing rate was fast. Instead of the normal "lub, dub" heart sounds he had a "gallop", sounding just like a horse racing by.

His ECG was normal but on heart ultrasound Unclassified Feline Cardiomyopathy was diagnosed with massive top heart chambers but relatively normal ventricles – so the rarest of cat heart muscle problems. Luckily, there was no evidence of internal clotting, known as thrombus formation. There was still some pericardial effusion but no evidence of remaining pleural effusion. With the owner's signed agreement, I added the drug combination of ACEI and Spironolactone, only licensed for dogs, that I had helped launch both on the Isle of Wight and elsewhere. Blue is doing brilliantly after his brush with the grim feline reaper.

So full retirement is in the distant future. I also planned a trip to Malawi for one last time under an African sky working for the World Veterinary Service. Sadly, COVID-19 (coronavirus disease 2019) has put paid to that. Yes, trip cancelled until humanity is rescued yet again by vaccination.

Today is Wednesday 3rd February 2021 and I have received my first dose of Pfizer COVID-19 vaccine on a day the UK had vaccinated 10 million of its 68 million population. I am also taking daily statins